The Molecular Control of Blood Cells

The Molecular Control of Blood Cells

Donald Metcalf

Harvard University Press
Cambridge, Massachusetts, and London, England   1988

Library of Congress Cataloging-in-Publication Data

Metcalf, Donald.
  The molecular control of blood cells / Donald Metcalf.
    p. cm.
  "Based on the Dunham lectures delivered in 1987 at
Harvard Medical School, Boston"—Pref.
  Bibliography: p.
  Includes index.
  ISBN 0-674-58157-1 (alk. paper)
  1. Hematopoiesis. 2. Colony-stimulating factors
  (Physiology).
I. Title. II. Title: Dunham lectures.
  [DNLM: 1. Blood Cells. 2. Colony-Stimulating
Factors—physiology. WH 140 M588m]
QP92.M484 1988
611'.0185—dc19
DNLM/DLC   88-605
for Library of Congress   CIP

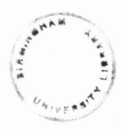

Preface

This book is based on the Dunham Lectures delivered in 1987 at Harvard Medical School, Boston. The lectures describe the exciting advances made in the past two decades in our knowledge, in molecular terms, of the control of normal and leukemic blood-forming cells.

I opened these lectures with the following quotation from Charles Darwin: "False facts are highly injurious to the progress of science, for they often long endure; but false views, if supported by some evidence do little harm, as everybody takes a salutary pleasure in proving their falseness." In describing our present knowledge of blood cell formation, I have followed the injunctions of Darwin by presenting as factual only a consensus of the observations of more than one group, but I have exercised some license in interpreting the implications of the observations.

At the request of Harvard University Press, I have written this book in a way that follows closely the form and spirit of the lectures; in particular, I have not provided exhaustive documentation of any of the statements made. To assist the reader, I have added a brief list of publications for further reading. These references should not be misconstrued as representing my view of what necessarily was the first or best piece of work on a certain subject. With their use, however, readers should be able to trace fairly quickly the original papers on each subject so, if need be, they can form an opinion regarding the validity and significance of the observations.

The unraveling of the complexities of the control of blood cell formation has been one of the most adventurous accomplishments in cell biology, and one that will have important consequences for the management of many serious human diseases. This book is dedicated to the many workers who have achieved these advances.

D.M.
Melbourne, Australia
November 1987

Contents

The Molecular Control of Blood Cells

1

The Basic Biology of Hemopoiesis

The cells circulating in the blood perform a variety of functions that are essential for survival of the organism. However, the blood cells and associated blood cell–forming (hemopoietic) tissue exhibit certain features which, in combination, make hemopoietic populations quite different from other vital organs in the body. These features include the short life span of mature blood cells, requiring continuous new blood cell formation throughout adult life; the multiplicity of blood cell types; and the wide dispersion of hemopoietic tissue in the body.

The number of new blood cells that the hemopoietic tissues must produce to replace effete cells is astonishingly large. In an adult human approximately 10^{10} red cells and 4×10^8 white cells are produced per hour. In normal health, levels of the various mature cells in the blood are maintained within quite narrow limits, yet in response to emergencies such as blood loss or infections, the hemopoietic tissues are able to respond rapidly by increasing cell production.

These considerations indicate that the regulation of hemopoiesis requires the existence of a quite complex control system. Fortunately, blood and hemopoietic cells are among the easiest cell populations to sample from an intact body; the cells possess a wealth of morphological and functional markers, and high-efficiency culture systems have been developed that allow much of hemopoiesis to be analyzed in vitro. With these advantages, a considerable body of information has been accumulated concerning the manner in which hemopoiesis is regulated.

This book will be concerned mainly with the mechanisms by which two closely related blood cell populations, granulocytes and macrophages, are controlled. The general principles emerging from this work are likely to apply also to other hemopoietic populations. What is less certain is how much of this information will be found to be applicable to other tissues in the body. Much of it may be of value in understanding the control of other tissues, but the hemopoietic tissues have often in the past been found to exhibit distinctive properties, and it may be that some aspects of their regulatory control systems are also quite novel.

The Hemopoietic Tissues

The mature cells in the peripheral blood of an animal are derived from eight distinct differentiation lineages—erythroid, neutrophil-granulocytic (hereafter referred to simply as granulocytic), monocytic, eosinophilic, mast cell, megakaryocytic, T-lymphoid, and B-lymphoid—together with some cells, such as natural killer cells, whose lineage remains unclear. The life spans of most of the mature cells of the different lineages are relatively short, ranging from a few days to a few months, although minor subpopulations of lymphoid cells can have a much longer life span.

Although none of these cells exhibits mitotic activity in the peripheral blood, it is a mistake to regard peripheral blood cells necessarily as end cells. Their potential for further proliferation varies widely, from absolutely zero in the case of nonnucleated erythroid cells and platelets, and probably zero in the case of mature granulocytes (polymorphs), to an extended potential capacity for proliferation in the case of monocytes, eosinophils, T-lymphocytes, and B-lymphocytes. The further proliferation of this last group of cells depends on their subsequent localization in the correct tissue and on activation by appropriate stimuli. Because most do not normally experience such circumstances, they behave, by default, as end cells.

The blood cells are best regarded as transit populations of cells that are destined to leave the circulation either to be destroyed or, less often, to enter a further phase in their life history in various tissue locations.

In an adult animal, the tissues generating the nonlymphoid cells of the peripheral blood are referred to as hemopoietic tissues and are restricted in location to the bone marrow and spleen. The vast bulk (more than 95 percent) of hemopoietic tissue is located in bone marrow in the form of scattered deposits in the cavities of bones such as the sternum, ribs, sacrum, vertebrae, and long bones.

Although this book will be concerned primarily with nonlymphoid populations, for completeness, a few words need to be added concerning the sites of formation of T-lymphocytes and B-lymphocytes. Most precursors of T-lymphocytes appear to arise in the bone marrow, but these cells must then seed in the thymus where expansion and differentiation of the T-lymphocyte population occur, with subsequent migration of a minor subset of these cells to peripheral organs such as the spleen and lymph nodes. Because some T-lymphocytes can be stimulated to undergo further extensive proliferation in the spleen and lymph nodes, the life history of individual T-lymphocytes can be quite complex.

A similar complexity applies to B-lymphocytes. In mammals most *de novo* formation of B-lymphocytes again occurs in the bone marrow, but in contrast to T-lymphocytes, considerable maturation of B-lymphocytes occurs in the marrow. However, B-lymphocytes also migrate to the spleen and lymph nodes, where amplification of B-lymphocyte populations can occur. It is also possible that some *de novo* formation of B-lymphocytes can occur in the spleen from resident stem cells. Thus newly formed T-lymphocytes or B-lymphocytes in the spleen or lymph nodes need not necessarily have originated from the bone marrow but may have been generated in one or another of the various peripheral lymphoid organs.

For the nonlymphoid blood cells the situation initially appeared to be simpler, with the marrow playing a dominant role and the spleen a minor (but extensible) role, and the two organs together being responsible for all new cell formation. However, more recent studies have emphasized the fact that mature monocytes, eosinophils, and mast cells need not necessarily be end cells; some can retain a potential for further proliferation. In normal health there is little evidence that these cells express this potential, but in abnormal states the situation can change and allow some local proliferation of these cells in nonhemopoietic tissues.

The Origin and Structure of the Hemopoietic Tissues

An unusual feature of the hemopoietic populations is that they originate from cells formed during embryogenesis as a discrete event of quite short duration. Early studies on the chicken and mouse indicated that the ancestral cells of hemopoietic tissue are generated in the yolk sac and then migrate into the developing liver of the embryo

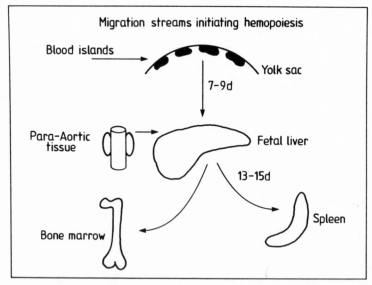

Figure 1. Origin of hemopoietic stem cells in yolk sac and dorsal mesentery and their sequential establishment of hemopoietic populations in the liver and then the marrow and spleen.

in a migration stream resembling that undertaken at the same time by gonadal germ cells to the developing gonads. These events occupy a brief period of only a few days; thereafter hemopoietic populations in the liver and subsequently in marrow and spleen are sustained and enlarged by the capacity of the original migrant hemopoietic stem cells for self-generation (Figure 1).

More recent studies, at least in the avian embryo, have indicated that these yolk sac–derived hemopoietic populations are in fact transient and are replaced by hemopoietic populations formed *de novo* in tissue in the para-aortic region of the dorsal mesentery. Although it is not yet clear whether this is true also for mammals, the second *de novo* formation of hemopoietic tissue is also finite in duration. Thus the hemopoietic tissues of the late fetus and the adult are forced to be self-sustaining and are maintained by the extended self-generative capacity of stem cells within the population. For this reason, a central problem to be resolved before the regulation of hemopoiesis can be fully understood is the manner in which stem cell self-generation is controlled.

After the initiation of hemopoietic populations in the yolk sac and/

or dorsal mesentery, the establishment of hemopoietic tissue in other organs occurs sequentially. The liver is the first organ to develop a hemopoietic population, and subsequently hemopoietic tissue appears in the developing bone marrow and spleen. With expansion of the marrow and spleen populations, the hemopoietic population in the liver declines shortly after birth. The liver then becomes a non-hemopoietic organ but retains a latent capacity to support hemopoiesis again in abnormal situations where both the marrow and spleen are damaged or diseased.

It is likely that the secondary establishment of hemopoietic populations in the marrow and spleen involves migration of stem cells from the liver population, but it is uncertain whether this secondary seeding continues for a prolonged period or tends also to be a brief episode with local self-generation of migrant stem cells dominating over continued stem cell migration.

The nonlymphoid hemopoietic tissues in a 25-g adult mouse total approximately 240×10^6 cells in the marrow and 10×10^6 cells in the spleen. Proliferative activity in these populations needs to replace at a rate of 2 percent per day the 12×10^9 red cells and a rate of 30 to 50 percent per day the 8×10^6 nonlymphoid cells in the peripheral blood. Thus the hemopoietic tissues need to generate cells approximately equal to their entire total number every day to replace existing blood cells.

In contrast to other organs such as the skin or gut, where extensive new cell production occurs throughout life, the hemopoietic tissues are not arranged in stratified layers of progressively more differentiated cells. Indeed, microscopic inspection of sections of marrow tissue suggests that the tissue is a random mixture of cells of different lineages and differentiation stages, with little evidence of either structural organization or segregation of cells of different lineages. This is not entirely true in all species, however; in the chicken, for example, there is some segregation of erythroid from granulocytic elements. Similarly, in the mouse spleen, granulocytic elements tend to be concentrated under the capsule and along the subcapsular trabeculae, whereas erythroid cells tend to be located in the red pulp itself. Furthermore, there is some evidence that the most ancestral hemopoietic cells (stem cells) may be concentrated at the periphery of the mouse marrow cavity.

Despite these minor segregations, the overwhelming impression remains that hemopoietic tissue is an unstructured mixture of cells of different lineages and differentiation stages.

The Clonal Nature of Hemopoiesis

The knowledge that hemopoietic populations are initiated and sustained by a relatively small number of stem cells immediately raises the possibility that these populations are in fact members of a quite limited number of clones initiated by these original stem cells. Indeed, most stem cells at any one time in adult life are noncycling, which also raises the possibility that hemopoiesis at any one time in adult life is being sustained by the proliferative activity of a quite restricted number of the available clonogenic stem cells.

These considerations lead to the expectation that, despite the lack of morphological evidence for stratification or segregation of hemopoietic populations, appropriate analysis of these populations should reveal clear evidence of hierarchical subsets of hemopoietic cells. Since clonally derived subpopulations of cells are a common feature of many tissues, it would be reasonable to anticipate the existence with hemopoietic populations of similar clonal subsets arranged in a descending hierarchy from stem cells to mature blood cells. This expectation has been confirmed experimentally by the development of in vivo and in vitro clonal assays that have documented the exis-

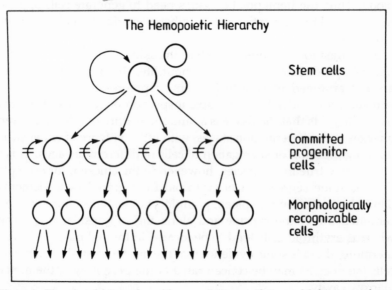

Figure 2. The clonal hierarchy of hemopoietic populations. Multipotential stem cells generate committed progenitor cells, which in turn generate morphologically identifiable cells that ultimately form the mature cells appearing in the blood. Each step involves a substantial amplification of cell numbers.

tence within hemopoietic populations of subsets of stem and progenitor cells with varying proliferative and differentiative capacity.

According to present knowledge, hemopoietic tissues can be represented as a series of functional compartments of increasing size, with individual cells in each compartment being able to generate variable numbers of progeny entering the next developmental compartment (Figure 2). Thus stem cells generate progenitor cells, which in turn generate morphologically identifiable progeny that progressively mature and ultimately lose their capacity for further proliferation, becoming the mature cells entering the blood.

This developmental sequence is characterized by certain phenomena:

1. The total number of progeny ultimately produced by any cell decreases with transit from one compartment to the next. Individual stem cells not only can self-generate but can produce progenitor cells each one of which can generate from 50 to 100,000 progeny. The immediate progeny of progenitor cells, for example myeloblasts or promyelocytes, generate smaller numbers of progeny, possibly only 2 to 200 in total.

2. Differentiation potential is similarly progressively reduced with transit from one compartment to the next. At least some stem cells can form all known types of hemopoietic and lymphoid cells. Progenitor cells, on the other hand, can be multipotential or bipotential but most commonly are unipotential, generating progeny of only a single differentiation lineage.

3. Stem cells can self-generate, but no other cells in the sequence possess this ability to any significant degree.

4. Cells cannot reverse the developmental sequence; for example, progenitor cells cannot form stem cells nor promyelocytes form progenitor cells.

5. Having undergone differentiation commitment in the progenitor cell compartment, individual cells cannot enter other differentiation lineages.

6. Within any one differentiation stage, considerable heterogeneity exists with respect to restriction of both proliferative and differentiative potential.

The techniques allowing this concept of hemopoiesis to be developed were as follows:

1. The development by Till and McCulloch in 1961 of an in vivo assay for stem cells based on the capacity of individual stem cells to form discrete hemopoietic colonies on the surface of the spleen when injected into lethally irradiated recipients.

2. The development by Bradley and Metcalf and by Pluznik and Sachs in the mid-1960s of clonal in vitro culture systems using semisolid medium. In these cultures individual progenitor cells and some stem cells can be identified by their capacity to generate colonies of maturing progeny.

3. The differential staining of maturing hemopoietic cells, allowing a likely sequence of maturation to be deduced from progressive changes in nuclear morphology and cytoplasmic structure—a creditable feat of careful observation and deductive logic by several generations of morphologists.

The experimental evidence supporting this current view of the interrelationships between the various hemopoietic populations will not be discussed in detail. Briefly, the key experimental observations documenting the validity of the model given above, shown schematically in Figure 3, are as follows:

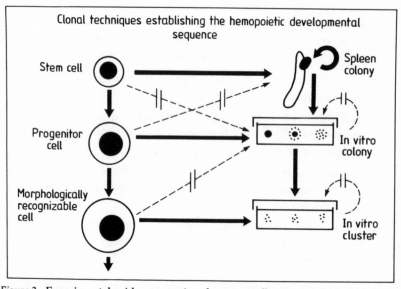

Figure 3. Experimental evidence proving that stem cells generate progenitor cells, which in turn generate morphologically identifiable hemopoietic cells.

1. Spleen colonies are generated by stem cells able to be separated by cell separation procedures as a distinct subset of hemopoietic cells. Spleen colonies generated by such cells themselves contain stem cells; this documents stem cell self-generation.

2. Spleen colonies contain progenitor cells; this documents the generation of progenitor cells from stem cells.

3. With few exceptions, purified progenitor cell populations cannot generate spleen colonies, and colonies grown in vitro from progenitor cells contain no stem cells and no progenitor cells; this documents an inability of cells to reverse the developmental sequence or of progenitor cells to self-generate.

4. In vitro colonies are clones and develop progressively maturing cells most often in a single differentiation lineage; this documents the production of morphologically identifiable and mature progeny by progenitor cells.

5. The frequency of stem and progenitor cells and their demonstrated, if variable, capacity to generate large numbers of progeny within a known time period are adequate to account for the required daily production of mature cells.

Hemopoiesis can therefore be represented graphically as the successive generation of clonally identifiable progeny with a progressive restriction of their proliferative and differentiative potential. The nomenclature applied to the various clonogenic cells is given in Figure 4.

Symmetry versus Asymmetry and the Nature of Stochastic Events in Hemopoiesis

The arrangement of hemopoietic tissue requires that stem cells be able both to self-generate and to generate differentiating progeny. This introduces a number of considerations, some of which are of the utmost importance for an appreciation of the fundamental abnormality in leukemic cells and indeed in all cancer cells.

A self-sustaining cell system that also continually produces progeny that ultimately die can maintain a constant population size only if half the progeny of the initiating clonogenic (stem) cells are themselves stem cells (self-generation). If fewer than 50 percent of the progeny of such stem cells are stem cells, the population will expend

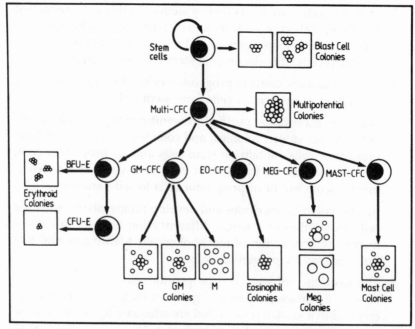

Figure 4. Schematic diagram of the stem and progenitor cells generating the mature blood cells, with their acronyms and a representation of the general features of the colonies formed in vitro by these cells.

itself unless renewed from some other source. For hemopoietic populations no such continuing extrinsic source exists, and the population of necessity must be self-supporting. Conversely, if more than 50 percent of progeny remain stem cell in nature, the total population will expand progressively—the basic situation in a cancer, since most cancers are the clonal progeny of a single initiating cell. Any attempted explanation of abnormal growth regulation in cancer or leukemia needs to recognize that, regardless of the abnormal balance of stimulatory versus inhibitory signals impinging on cancer stem cells, the crucial intrinsic abnormality in the cancer cell is its inappropriate response to signaling resulting in an imbalance during cell division favoring self-generation. This is a seemingly self-evident proposition, but one that is somewhat difficult to accept in cases where stem cells may constitute only a quite small fraction of an established tumor or leukemic population. It must be appreciated that the relative size of the stem versus other, often differentiating, populations in a cancer depends on the fate or life span of the non–stem

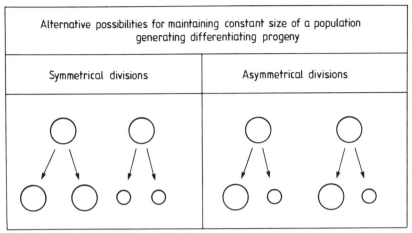

Figure 5. Two methods by which immature cells (*large circles*) can generate differentiating progeny (*small circles*): *left panel*, by symmetrical divisions; *right panel*, by asymmetrical divisions.

cell population, and the relative numbers of the two populations are a parameter that gives by itself no valid indication of the behavior of the stem cells.

There are two different ways in which stem cells could divide and maintain constant stem cell numbers (Figure 5): by *symmetrical division*, where on average half the stem cells produce progeny cells both of which are themselves stem cells, and half the stem cells produce progeny that enter an irreversible differentiation sequence; or by *asymmetrical division*, where each stem cell generates two daughters, one of which is a stem cell while the other enters a differentiation sequence. This same question can be posed repeatedly throughout the various differentiation stages in hemopoiesis. For example, does a myeloblast form one myeloblast and one promyelocyte, or do alternate myeloblasts produce two myeloblasts or two promyelocytes?

The basic question of symmetry versus asymmetry has proved very difficult to resolve in any cell system. However, there are now observations on developing nematodes and on individual cultured hemopoietic cells to indicate that asymmetrical divisions certainly do occur and, at least in hemopoietic populations, are likely to be the usual type.

This raises as a fundamental issue the cellular mechanisms responsible for the occurrence of asymmetrical divisions, and the question of whether the process is immutable or can be modulated by external

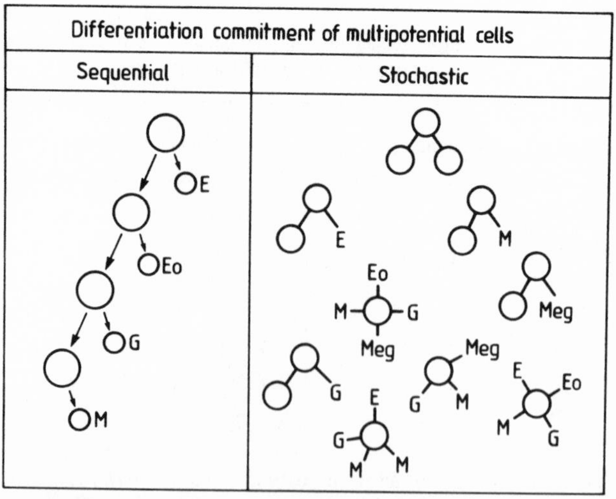

Figure 6. Two methods by which multipotential cells might generate unipotential progeny. The left panel shows the generation of unipotential progeny in a fixed sequence; the right panel shows the generation of unipotential progeny occurring as a random (stochastic) series of events.

Is signalling intrinsic of stem cells?

signaling. In light of the earlier comments regarding the essential abnormality in cancer cells, it becomes a question of major practical importance to establish whether abnormally high levels of self-generation can be suppressed by manipulating extrinsic signals impinging on a cell.

Analysis of several hemopoietic systems has clearly indicated that asymmetry in self-renewal is stochastic in nature (Figure 6). This has best been documented by the in vitro analysis of commitment of multipotential and bipotential cells entering one or more of a number of available differentiation lineages. What has caused considerable confusion to some has been the misconception that the random (stochastic) nature of these processes indicates that the processes are immutable. There is, of course, nothing of this nature implicit in a stochastic event. Although self-generation by stem cells is a stochastic process, this self-generation occurs with a certain probability (P), and the value of P is not necessarily constant and immutable. When stem cells are forced to generate a spleen colony or to regenerate the hemopoietic tissue of an animal in which the preexisting population has been destroyed by irradiation or cytotoxic drugs, not only does the population of maturing cells increase but also, for a time, the relative frequency of stem cells. Clearly in this situation, the P value for self-generation must for a time have been increased. Later, in Chapter 10, an example will be discussed where the P value for leukemic stem cell self-generation can be reduced essentially to zero by the action of a normal regulator molecule.

The conclusions to be drawn from these observations are that asymmetry is a fundamental aspect of the behavior of normal and leukemic hemopoietic cells and that, although this appears to be a stochastic process, the probability of self-generative versus differentiative divisions can be altered. The mechanisms controlling this process are largely unknown and remain one of the major outstanding problems to be solved in the attempt to elucidate the control of hemopoiesis.

Hemopoietic Stem Cells

The key cells in sustaining hemopoiesis are the multipotential hemopoietic stem cells. Although these cells can be enumerated by the use of the spleen colony assay, they constitute an exceedingly small fraction (approximately 0.2 percent) of the total hemopoietic population even during active regeneration of hemopoietic tissues. If one traces hemopoiesis back to its initiation in the yolk sac, *all* the original hemopoietic cells were likely to have been stem cells, whereas even in the early developing fetal liver the frequency of stem cells is already low.

Use of the spleen colony technique was successful in establishing certain basic properties of stem cells: (1) their ability to generate clonally expanding populations of maturing cells, (2) their ability to undergo extensive self-generation, (3) their multipotentiality, and (4) the fact that most stem cells in an adult are not in cell cycle. These in vivo studies also produced evidence that at least some individual stem cells could generate both hemopoietic and lymphoid progeny.

Further progress in characterizing stem cells was impeded by two problems: the low frequency of stem cells, which prevented their ready morphological identification, and the cumbersome nature of the in vivo assay system. Stem cells were eventually purified by fluorescence-activated cell sorting, initially using rat cells where the uniquely high Thy-1 antigen expression on stem cells allowed a relatively easy series of separative procedures. The morphology of the stem cell in the rat and other species is that of a medium-sized mononuclear cell with prominent nucleoli and a narrow rim of slightly basophilic agranular cytoplasm. For the morphologist, the tempting description of these cells is "lymphocyte-like"—an accurate enough morphological description, but extremely unfortunate in its connotation because stem cells are quite distinct from any bona fide lymphocyte population.

Purified stem cells have been used to generate typical spleen colonies, eliminating an early possibility that several injected cell types might need to interact to generate a spleen colony. This latter possibility was the basis for the original name for stem cells of colony-forming unit-spleen (CFU-S).

More recent studies on stem cells have documented the extreme heterogeneity of cells classifiable in this category because of their ability to generate spleen colonies. This heterogeneity seems to be twofold in nature: a proliferative history-based hierarchy in which certain cells with a previous history of extensive cell division now express a relatively restricted capacity for further self-generation or progeny generation, and a differentiation-based heterogeneity in which cells may still retain some capacity for self-generation but have lost one or more differentiative capacities—for example, are now only capable of generating granulocytes and erythroid cells but not lymphoid or megakaryocytic progeny.

The more closely individual stem cells are examined, the more evident it becomes that scarcely any two stem cells are absolutely identical in proliferative and differentiative potentiality. Indeed, it may be that, if sufficiently stringent tests were to be applied, the concept of absolute self-generative capacity might have to be abandoned because progeny stem cells at the very least have undergone one further cell division than the parent.

At a more practical level, the obvious heterogeneity in stem cells has allowed a case to be made for distinguishing three broad classes of stem cells: (1) cells with an exceptional proliferative and self-generative capacity, which are called by some "repopulating cells" and are held to be the cells in a marrow transplant that are ultimately responsible for repopulating a depleted recipient and establishing a persisting hemopoietic population; (2) day 14 CFU-S, cells with extensive self-renewal and proliferative capacity forming spleen colonies observable at day 14 in irradiated recipients; and (3) day 7 CFU-S, cells with a more restricted capacity for self-renewal and proliferation forming transient colonies observable at day 7. The issues raised by this subdivision are, first, whether a distinct compartment of repopulating cells exists that is the only population of real relevance in sustaining hemopoiesis or repopulation, and second, to what degree day 7 CFU-S cells overlap with or are identical to the multipotential colony-forming cells able to be grown in semisolid cultures. These issues are of practical importance for those trying to optimize marrow transplantation in the clinical setting. If the three subsets of stem cells represent merely a continuous spectrum within the rather heterogeneous stem cell population, then potentially all are of value when transplanted. If repopulating cells are a distinct subpopulation, however, then any separative procedures used prior to transplantation must ensure that these cells are preserved.

Recently it has been recognized that at least some stem cells are able to form colonies in semisolid cultures. Whether repopulating cells can form such colonies is unclear, but evidence has been obtained that cells from at least some in vitro colonies can repopulate irradiated recipients. At present, the culture systems used to grow stem cell colonies also support the growth of larger and more numerous colonies derived from progenitor cells. This makes it extremely difficult to work with stem cell colonies in vitro. However, if available improved cell separation techniques are used to separate stem from progenitor cells, the ability to culture purified stem cells in vitro should greatly simplify efforts to determine the factors controlling the proliferation and self-generation of these cells.

Hemopoietic Progenitor Cells

Progenitor cells, or committed progenitor cells, are the immediate progeny of stem cells. Their detection and characterization as a class were made possible by the introduction of semisolid clonal cultures in which individual progenitor cells can be detected because of their ability to generate colonies of differentiating progeny.

The original clonal culture system identified progenitor cells able to form colonies of granulocytes and/or macrophages. The most important conclusion from this early work was that neutrophilic granulocytes and monocyte-macrophages are closely related populations, in many cases sharing the same common progenitor cell. Subsequent work has developed comparable in vitro clonal cultures permitting enumeration of all other types of progenitor cells (see Figure 4).

Analysis of colonies generated in vitro by progenitor cells established the following information regarding this type of cell: (1) colonies are clones generated by single progenitor cells; different progenitor cells have the capacity to produce varying numbers of progeny from 50 to 10^5 cells within a 7- to 10-day period; (2) the most frequent colonies are of a single lineage, and thus the most numerous progenitors are unipotential cells precommitted to one differentiation lineage; (3) most colonies contain no stem cells and no progenitor cells; thus progenitor cells can neither reverse the developmental sequence nor self-generate; (4) with time, colony cells exhibit reasonably complete differentiation to fully mature cells; thus this process does not of necessity require cell-to-cell contact with other cells; (5) unlike stem cells, most progenitor cells in the adult animal are in active cell cycle; (6) the total frequency of all types of progenitor cells in an adult hemopoietic population is low (approximately 1 percent of total cells).

As was the case with stem cells, progress in identifying progenitor cells hinged on removing contaminating cells by cell-sorting procedures, particularly in the use of fluorescence-activated cell sorting. Progenitor cells are medium- to large-sized blast cells with cytoplasm that is basophilic and without cytoplasmic granules.

From the outset, it was obvious that progenitor cells were likely to be highly heterogeneous. There is a wide variation in morphology, size, and differentiative state between different hemopoietic colonies growing in vitro in the same culture dish. Even with colonies of any one morphological type (for example, erythroid or macrophage), this same extreme range is observable. Heterogeneity is clearly evident in every separative procedure used to analyze progenitor cells, for example, adherence, density, size, charge, or surface antigens. The biological basis for this heterogeneity is essentially similar to that responsible for stem cell heterogeneity: differences in proliferative past history and consequent future proliferative potential and differences based on differentiation precommitment.

It was postulated for a time by certain researchers that only a single class of progenitor cell exists, and that irreversible differentiation commitment occurs following contact of a particular regulatory molecule with such cells. This proposal would have been tenable only if all progenitor cells express membrane receptors for all possible regulatory molecules. In fact, progenitor cells do indeed co-express receptors for more than one type of regulatory molecule, but the single-population hypothesis seemed improbable in view of the widely differing physical characteristics of progenitor cells. Formal proof of the existence of distinct subsets of precommitted progenitor cells has been surprisingly difficult to obtain even using a wide variety of monoclonal antisera and other membrane probes. There are still no separative techniques that can obtain a purified population of erythroid or other lineage-restricted progenitor cells. However, there are now numerous studies in which clear, if incomplete, segregation has been achieved of various progenitor cell subsets, making it virtually certain that lineage-committed subsets of committed progenitor cells do exist.

As in the case of stem cells, at the extreme ends of the progenitor cell range these populations tend to merge with preceding and succeeding populations. Thus progenitors exist that are capable of generating colonies containing erythroid, granulocytic, macrophage, eosinophil, and megakaryocytic progeny, and at least some of these contain progenitor cells and cells able to generate at least day 7 spleen colonies. Such multipotential progenitor cells clearly approach the criteria categorizing the more mature stem cells.

At the other extreme are clonogenic cells that outnumber progenitor cells in frequency but are capable of generating clones only of restricted size, for example, the CFU-E generating small erythroid colonies and the cluster-forming cells generating clones of subcolony size in other lineages. Such cells are the immediate progeny of more ancestral progenitor cells and in turn merge with those morphologically identifiable cells retaining some capacity for further limited proliferation. Thus human promyelocytes are readily identifiable morphologically but are also capable of generating small, transient, granulocytic clones in vitro, some of which can achieve the lower size limit required of human colonies (40 cells).

It is predictable that, given good or artificially enhanced culture conditions, any cell capable of even one division can be detected as proliferating in vitro. Such cultures can have valuable uses, but to classify cells generating minute clones as progenitor cells has little value.

Summary

The hemopoietic tissues constitute a complex, self-sustaining population that continuously generates maturing cells in multiple differentiation lineages. Despite an absence of architectural stratification, hemopoietic populations have been shown by clonal analysis to contain a hierarchy of ancestral clonogenic cells, the most important of which are the multipotential stem cells and their immediate progeny, lineage-restricted committed progenitor cells. Cells within both of these populations exhibit considerable heterogeneity with respect to physical characteristics, as well as proliferative and differentiative potential.

The arrangement of hemopoietic subpopulations requires the existence not only of mechanisms controlling cell proliferation but also of mechanisms controlling self-generative versus differentiative cell divisions and for inducing differentiation commitment.

2

*General Aspects of the
Control of Hemopoiesis*

In normal health, levels of the various blood cells are maintained within reasonably narrow limits. Based on the distribution of hemopoietic cells, the general requirements of a control system for this population are, first, that the proliferative activity of aggregates of hemopoietic tissue in widely scattered locations must be closely controlled and coordinated, and second, at the same time the system must be able to respond rapidly to changing needs in emergency situations such as blood loss, acute infections, or following exposure to cytotoxic agents.

Since the other tissues in the body depend for their survival on the functional activity of the blood cells, the most logical control system would be one in which the dependent tissues were capable of monitoring actual blood cell levels and, if necessary, initiating signals modulating cell production (a demand-control system). This is easiest to visualize in the case of red cells, whose major function is oxygen transport. Sensor cells, if distributed in all organs, could respond to changes in oxygen tension; then under anoxic conditions, these cells could synthesize and release to the circulation a specific molecule initiating additional red cell production. The advantage of such a system is that a humoral regulator could best cope with the problem of regulating overall cell proliferation by widely dispersed hemopoietic tissues. Indeed, the first observation relating to the control of hemopoiesis was the discovery in 1906 by Carnot and Deflandre of a factor in anemic serum, erythropoietin, able to stimulate red cell formation.

Comparable demand-generated regulatory systems could be envisaged for other blood cells, such as the release by damaged endothelial cells of a stimulus for megakaryoctye proliferation and the formation of platelets needed to repair the damage or the production by tissues damaged by bacterial infection of factors able to stimulate the formation of granulocytes, monocytes, or eosinophils.

In this simplest type of control system, cessation of demand would terminate the state of increased signaling for proliferation and allow cell production to return to basal levels. However, mathematical modeling of such an arrangement has suggested the need for associated inhibitory signals to avoid the system being subject to progressive cyclical fluctuations.

If specific progenitor cells existed that were able to respond selectively to stimulation by a particular regulatory molecule, a demand-regulated humoral control system would also be able to achieve another desirable requirement of a control system—that the proliferative response be selective and involve only the appropriate subpopulation of hemopoietic cells. However, as discussed in the previous chapter, progenitor cells are essentially a transit population with no capacity for self-maintenance; consequently, to achieve sustained responses, a mechanism is also needed for regulating the production of new progenitor cells from stem cells. If stem cells exhibit receptors for all known regulatory molecules (a point not yet established), the same signal molecule, for example, erythropoietin, regulating the production of maturing red cells could also be envisaged as being able to stimulate erythroid progenitor cell formation from stem cells. The potential problem presented by such an arrangement is that if progenitor cell commitment to different lineages is a stochastic and unmodulatable process, a signal such as erythropoietin initiating stem cell proliferation to generate additional erythroid progenitors would be inefficient because it would involve the unnecessary and wasteful formation of other hemopoietic progenitors.

In this context the simple bleeding of an animal, which provokes increased erythropoiesis, has in fact been observed to elevate the numbers of granulocyte-macrophage progenitors, and there may well be some inefficiency in the manner in which the demand for additional specific progenitor cells is met. However, the major objection to this proposed erythropoietin-based control system is the observation that, at least for mouse cells, erythropoietin can stimulate neither the proliferation of the most immature erythroid progenitors nor that of stem cells. It is therefore clear that, in the case of erythroid cell formation, a single regulator molecule is not sufficient to achieve the desired increased erythropoiesis; either additional humoral regulators are required, or some additional type of control system is involved.

It is possible, of course, to propose systems other than the demand-control system by which the level of production of humoral regulators might be modulated. One proposal receiving some attention is that the hemopoietic populations might be internally self-regulating, with either stimulatory or inhibitory humoral regulators being the exclusive products of mature hemopoietic cells. Alternatively, other tissues could produce such factors in response to monitoring secretion or breakdown products of mature blood cells. The general problem with control systems based solely on the *levels* of mature cells is that they cannot explain how regeneration can be achieved following depletion of the populations while at the same time permitting the sustained overproduction of mature cells when necessary.

What is no longer possible to postulate is that hemopoietic cells in fact require no positive stimulation for proliferation and that the only control system required is a series of inhibitory regulators. Observations on the growth of granulocyte-macrophage colonies and subsequently on colonies of other types indicated that stem and progenitor cells are not capable of spontaneous, or self-stimulated, cell division. Unless in vitro cultures are quite misleading in this regard, these observations eliminate all hypotheses regarding hemopoietic cell control in which cell division occurs as an inevitable consequence of the cells being alive and having access to adequate nutritional metabolites.

Theoretical consideration of the problem to be solved in hemopoietic regulation therefore predicts the existence of multiple specific humoral regulatory molecules. However, much of the work on hemopoiesis done in the 1960s using the spleen colony-forming technique suggested that hemopoiesis was somehow controlled by local microenvironmental cells adjacent to, or within, foci of hemopoietic cells.

A number of observations led to this general conclusion:

1. Although stem cells are present in the blood and could seed in any organ, in fact hemopoiesis is restricted to two tissues, the marrow and the spleen, suggesting some special requirement provided by these sites.

2. Spleen colonies early in development most often appear to contain cells of only one differentiation lineage, while adjacent colonies may contain cells of a quite different lineage. This observation led to the hypothesis that perhaps physical spaces existed that were bounded by specialized cells that committed

entering stem cells to one or another lineage and possibly then supported their subsequent proliferation.

3. Three additional observations appeared to support this hypothesis. Colonies in the spleen of an irradiated recipient most often were composed of differentiating erythroid cells, whereas comparable colonies in the marrow most often were granulocytic in composition. If a bone shaft was implanted in the spleen and a colony, by chance, developed at the shaft-spleen interface, the spleen portion was composed of erythroid cells while the marrow portion contained granulocytes. Similarly, as spleen colonies expanded, second populations of maturing cells of another lineage developed, but these tended to be segregated to the margin of the colony. Thus an expanding erythroid colony might develop a peripheral focus of granulocytic cells, suggesting that an uncommitted stem cell from the erythroid colony had entered an adjacent granulocytic niche (Figure 7).

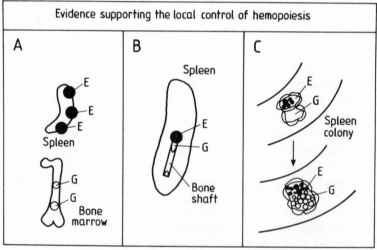

Figure 7. Key evidence from hemopoietic colony formation in irradiated recipients supporting the concept of local control of differentiation commitment of stem cells. *(A)* Colonies in the spleen tend to be erythroid (E), while those in the marrow are granulocytic (G). *(B)* Colonies at the interface of a bone shaft implanted in the spleen are erythroid in the spleen half but granulocytic in the marrow half. *(C)* Expanding spleen colonies develop second populations at the periphery, consistent with entry of a colony stem cell into an adjacent (granulocytic) niche.

This compelling morphological evidence from clonal hemopoiesis in vivo needs some reappraisal in the light of subsequent studies analyzing in vitro the composition of individual spleen colonies. Although most early spleen colonies appear to contain only maturing erythroid cells, they in fact also contain a wide range of committed progenitors of other lineages, for example, granulocytic, monocytic, eosinophilic, or megakaryocytic. As a result, it is difficult to sustain the hypothesis that lineage-specific niches exist in which unipotential commitment occurs. Within spleen colonies the generation of progenitor cells appears, at least superficially, to be a stochastic process leading rather indiscriminately to the generation of all types of progenitors. The obvious preponderance of differentiating cells of one lineage within a colony must therefore be due to subsequent events, and it remains reasonable to postulate that the microenvironment cells of the specialized niche could be sources of short-range specific growth factors (for example, for erythroid cells) or could achieve the same result by displaying on their membranes lineage-specific growth factor molecules. Either process would achieve the selective clonal expansion of one hemopoietic subpopulation and account for the observed characteristics of spleen colony formation.

Powerful supporting evidence for a vital role played by hemopoietic stromal or microenvironmental cells in regulating hemopoiesis has come from culture studies using adherent layers of stromal cells derived from marrow populations (the Dexter culture technique). In these cultures, stem cell self-generation is maintained over long periods, the concentration of stem cells being highest within the underlayer itself. Furthermore, such cultures sustain for long periods the production of progenitor cells of multiple types as well as differentiating progeny of these cells. Morphological examination of such cultures has produced clear evidence of the focal generation of hemopoietic cells in islets attached to the underlayer cells, particularly around cells that have undergone lipid accumulation.

These observations strongly suggest that certain stromal cells can play a vital role in controlling hemopoiesis and that they do so by intimate cell contact, again raising possibilities of membrane-displayed molecules or the secretion of short-range molecules.

More recent studies have succeeded in isolating cloned cell lines from such marrow stromal cells, some of which display an impressive capacity to support stem and progenitor cell proliferation most clearly by a cell contact process. Unfortunately, studies on some cell lines derived from nonhemopoietic tissues, for example, fibroblasts, have also demonstrated their ability to support cell-contact hemopoiesis. If indeed fibroblasts from many locations can support complex hemopoietic events in vitro, this leaves a rather unsatisfactory situation in which the selective initiation of hemopoiesis in the marrow and spleen may no longer be able to be explained satisfactorily.

A final phenomenon should be mentioned relating to the control of hemopoiesis by stromal underlayers. Studies using certain of these cloned stromal cell lines have documented that they can modulate the responses of hemopoietic cells to humoral regulatory molecules, for example, modifying the proportion of self-generative versus differentiative cell divisions.

Despite the impressive morphological evidence linking the control of stem and progenitor cell formation with adjacent stromal cells, there is now clear evidence from the clonal in vitro culture of single stem or multipotential cells that the generation of these cells does not require the mandatory presence of hemopoietic stromal cells. Single stem cells can generate colonies containing both stem and progenitor cells if appropriate stimulating factors are added to the cultures. Furthermore, it is not uncommon in colonies grown in vitro from single multipotential cells for a dramatic segregation of cell types to be observed, with erythroid cells in one half of the colony and nonerythroid cells in the other—a major keystone in the evidence supporting the specialized niche hypothesis.

An obvious possibility that would unify both the niche hypothesis and the clonal culture observations is that both sets of observations have the same molecular basis. In the one case, the regulatory molecules are displayed on the membranes of stromal cells, while in culture these molecules have been presented in soluble form. However, given the complexity of molecular regulation of hemopoietic cells that is now apparent, this unifying proposal is also likely to be too simple; it is likely that some regulatory molecules displayed on stromal cells are unique to certain cell types and are never secreted as humoral molecules.

Summary

Earlier models of hemopoietic control systems postulated that the stem cell to progenitor cell step might be controlled by cell contact or short-range interactions with specialized stromal cells, while the production of differentiating progeny might be regulated by humoral

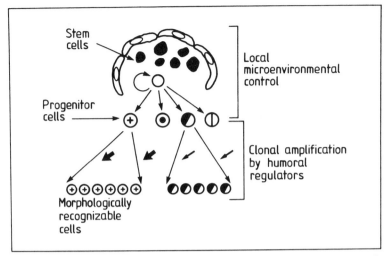

Stem cells

Progenitor cells

Local microenvironmental control

Clonal amplification by humoral regulators

Morphologically recognizable cells

Figure 8. Diagrammatic representation of the control of blood cell formation. Stem cells generate progenitor cells under regulation by microenvironmental cells. The clonal production of maturing cells from progenitor cells is regulated by specific humoral regulators.

regulatory molecules (Figure 8). This two-stage model no longer seems valid; a better view is to propose that both types of control system operate at all levels, possibly with some bias favoring stem cell control by stromal cells and a more important role of humoral regulators in later developmental stages.

In the following chapter on the humoral control of granulocyte-macrophage populations, the underlying complexity of the complete control systems must be kept in mind. At the present stage it has been technically simpler to identify and characterize humoral regulators, but it would be naive to expect that these molecules alone are sufficient to regulate in the most efficient manner even the relatively simple process of the formation of maturing cells from committed granulocyte-macrophage progenitor cells.

3

The Colony-Stimulating Factors
and Their Receptors

From the discussion in the preceding chapter of ways in which the hemopoietic population might be regulated, the existence of a set of specific positive humoral regulators stands out as almost mandatory, since these would best meet the peculiar requirements of a system in which tissues throughout the body need to signal the necessity for the production of new cells to widely dispersed collections of hemopoietic tissue.

The first such humoral regulator, erythropoietin, was discovered in the serum as early as 1906 using a quite simple animal model. At the time it must have seemed a relatively simple matter to extend this work and detect comparable regulators for other blood cells. However, the next 60 years elapsed without the discovery of additional regulators other than a rather ill-defined factor, thrombopoietin, which was able to produce some elevation of platelet levels. In retrospect, the numerous attempts in this period to detect other regulators probably failed for two reasons. First, other blood cells have a more complex life history in the intact animal, making it more difficult to detect small perturbations in the production of the relevant hemopoietic subpopulations. Second, it is now known that the concentrations of regulators in the blood and tissues are extremely low, and their detection in such concentrations requires the use of highly sensitive in vitro assay systems.

Beginning in the mid-1960s, with the introduction of the semisolid culture techniques able to support the proliferation of the various types of hemopoietic cells in vitro, this situation changed; in the following twenty years specific regulators for all blood cell subsets were detected and characterized. Since the advent of molecular biol-

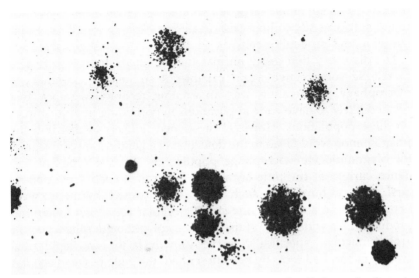

Figure 9. Murine granulocyte-macrophage colonies after 7 days of culture in semisolid medium.

ogy into this field in the last four years, the pace of discovery has increased at an astonishing rate.

This chapter will be concerned mainly with the discovery and characterization of the specific molecules controlling granulocyte-macrophage production and function, because more is known about these molecules than about some of the others, and they serve as useful models exemplifying the peculiarities of these regulators. It seems likely that most of the features of these molecules and the questions they raise will apply equally to the currently less well characterized regulators of other hemopoietic subpopulations.

During the analysis of the original clonal culture technique for granulocyte-macrophage colonies, it was noted that the culture of mouse marrow or spleen cell suspensions alone did not result in colony formation. On the other hand, if underlayers containing various cells or tissue fragments were inserted under the cultures, prominent granulocyte-macrophage colonies developed (Figure 9). The conclusion reached was that granulocyte-macrophage precursors (eventually identified as progenitor cells) were unable to proliferate in otherwise satisfactory culture medium unless the cells were stimulated. This conclusion—that granulocyte-macrophage progenitors are not capable of spontaneous or self-stimulated cell division—has been found subsequently to hold true as a generalization for all hemopoietic stem and progenitor cells.

The discovery that many normal and neoplastic tissues were able to release some active agent capable of stimulating granulocyte-macrophage proliferation was an exciting technical advance that seemed likely to have wide applications in permitting in vitro studies on these populations. However, it seemed unlikely at first that the phenomenon would lead to the detection of a genuine specific regulator of granulocyte-macrophage populations. Several types of evidence current at the time seemed to be against such a possibility. First, classical hormones, such as insulin or growth hormone, were known to have a single, quite specific cellular source and were not produced by a wide range of tissues. Second, although other types of growth factors, specifically nerve growth factor and epidermal growth factor, had recently been described, the wide range of cellular sources of these factors was not yet appreciated. Third, Puck and his colleagues had introduced the proposal that single cells (fibroblasts) had difficulty proliferating in vitro because of diffusion of low-molecular-weight metabolites from the cultured cell into the medium. The flow of such vital metabolites was postulated to be corrected by the addition of large numbers of filler or feeder cells, which would diffuse such metabolites and thus reverse the diffusion gradient. Certainly, this maneuver permitted single cells to remain viable and capable of division. Finally, in the early 1960s, based on the behavior of normal fibroblasts versus sarcoma cells, it was believed that only transformed cells were able to proliferate in agar culture (the semisolid medium used for growing granulocyte-macrophage colonies). If this conclusion held true also for granulocytes and macrophages, colony formation by granulocyte-macrophage cells was likely to have been the consequence of some transformation event that had occurred during the culture period.

This accumulated evidence tended to create a somewhat pessimistic view of the possible value of using the granulocyte-macrophage colony-forming technique to detect specific regulators of granulocyte-macrophage populations, the more so because information from animal studies had suggested that a wide range of injected materials could alter levels of white blood cells, particularly granulocytes. Although the cells in granulocyte-macrophage colonies appeared to differentiate during culture to recognizable mature cells, the greatest single worry, at least in our laboratory at the Hall Institute, was that some virus might have transformed the cultured cells, particularly since the original methods used to stimulate granulocyte-macrophage colony formation were the addition of cells or serum from mice with lymphoid leukemia. With the technology available 20 years ago, it was not a simple matter to distinguish between viruses and protein macromolecules as the agent involved in a particular phenomenon.

Because of these uncertainties regarding the possible lack of specificity of the phenomenon and the possible involvement of viruses, much of our initial work at the Hall Institute on granulocyte-macrophage colony formation involved the gathering of indirect evidence that would support the notion that the active factor (given the operational name of *colony-stimulating factor* or *CSF*) was likely to be a genuine regulator molecule. The following preliminary studies were performed:

1. Attempts were made to eliminate the possible involvement of viruses by the use of normal tissues, studies using viral inactivation by ultraviolet light, or physical separative methods to eliminate viruses from serum or medium conditioned by active tissues.

2. Detectable CSF was searched for in the serum and urine, particularly those of normal animals and humans.

3. Evidence was sought that serum or urine CSF levels fluctuated appropriately in conditions where perturbations in granulocyte-macrophage populations were occurring in vivo, for example, during infections.

4. Evidence was sought that various normal tissues contained and/or produced detectable amounts of CSF, in concentrations, it was hoped, exceeding those in the serum.

The logic behind this approach was that if a candidate regulator was indeed of genuine significance in vivo, then it should be detectable in the serum and tissues in concentrations adequate to stimulate cell proliferation in vitro, and, given the lability of granulocyte-macrophage levels in vivo under abnormal conditions, a similar variability in regulator levels should be demonstrable.

This survey approach occupied five years but did establish a firm presumptive case that CSF was likely to be a genuine regulator of granulocyte-macrophage populations in vivo. The findings were as follows:

1. CSF was detectable in low levels in the serum of mice and humans and in normal human urine.

2. CSF levels were elevated in the serum and urine of animals and patients with acute infections due to viruses or bacteria (Figure 10) and in animals and patients with some forms of advanced cancer where secondary infections were possible.

3. Serum CSF levels were low or undetectable in germ-free animals but became elevated following conventionalization.

4. Damage to hemopoietic populations by irradiation or cytotoxic drugs led to elevations in serum CSF levels in conventional animals but not in germ-free animals.

5. CSF was extractable from all major tissues in the mouse, and in concentrations higher than in the serum.

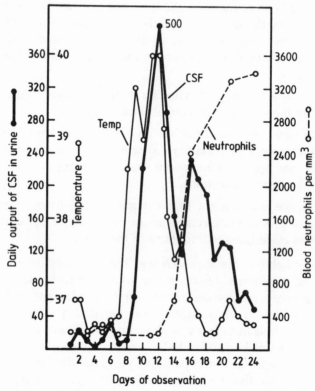

Figure 10. Rise in CSF levels in the urine of a patient with acute myeloid leukemia during an episode of septicemia. Levels of urinary CSF returned to normal after control of the infection.

6. Serum CSF levels were elevated dramatically by the injection of endotoxin, bacterial antigens, and certain other foreign proteins. Tissue levels of CSF also rose following the injection of endotoxin.

Purification of the CSFs

With this background of supporting evidence, it was felt reasonable in our laboratories at the Hall Institute to expend a major effort on the purification of CSF even though, in light of the data then emerging from studies on the purification of erythropoietin, this was likely to be a formidable project because of the low concentrations of the active factor.

The commitment to begin purification of CSF involved making a difficult decision regarding the choice of a starting material. This type of decision has remained a constant dilemma throughout all subsequent work on hemopoietic regulators until the advent of molecular biology and the ability sometimes to use expression screening of cDNA libraries as a direct approach to isolating rare molecules. In essence, the dilemma involves a choice between two alternative types of source material. In the first place cell lines, often neoplastic, may be producing relatively high levels of the factor often in serum-free medium, whereas normal tissues often produce far lower levels of active material. The first type of source is obviously superior for technical reasons that include the ability to mass-produce the starting material and to use low concentrations of serum in the cultures. The risk involved, however, is that the cells are likely to be highly abnormal and either may not be producing a normal factor or may be producing it in a quite abnormal form.

By the early 1970s it was known that L-cells and comparable cultures of uncharacterized embryo cells were a rich source of CSF; this led to what proved to be a successful series of purification studies, resulting first in highly enriched CSF and finally purified CSF. At the Hall Institute we chose to adopt the less favorable alternative of using normal starting materials, initially using normal human urine as a cheap and readily available source material and later using medium conditioned by lung tissue from mice injected by endotoxin, since this tissue was clearly superior to others in its ability to produce CSF in culture (Figure 11).

As the studies in various laboratories progressed in parallel, it became increasingly obvious that the situation with CSF was more com-

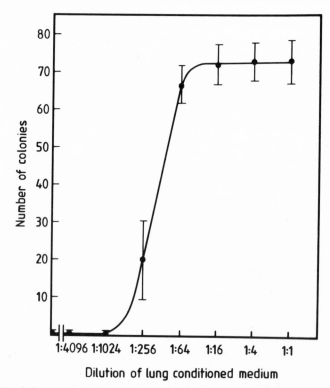

Figure 11. Colony-stimulating activity of medium conditioned by lung tissue from mice preinjected with endotoxin. Subsequent studies showed that this medium contains a mixture of GM-CSF and G-CSF.

plex than originally envisaged from the only existing model, erythropoietin:

1. The CSF produced by L-cells and embryo cell lines appeared to be a glycoprotein of quite large size (molecular weight approximately 70,000), and the colonies stimulated were mainly macrophage in composition, unlike the mixture of granulocytic and macrophage colonies stimulated by the original tissue underlayers or conditioned medium from such tissues.

2. CSF purified from human urine exhibited distinct differences. It did stimulate macrophage colony formation by mouse bone marrow cells, but the CSF appeared to be a smaller glycoprotein of molecular weight 45,000. Moreover, with the introduction of a modified culture technique supporting granulocyte-macrophage colony formation by human cells, it was disconcerting

that human urinary CSF had little or no proliferative effect on human cells.

3. The CSF produced by mouse lung tissue appeared to be functionally quite different in that it stimulated granulocyte and/or macrophage colony formation, resembling that seen originally with the early underlayer experiments. Further, although this CSF was also a glycoprotein, its molecular weight was 23,000, much smaller than the two known forms from mouse L-cells or human urine.

4. Extensive studies on the nature of the CSFs produced in vitro by eight different mouse tissues showed that the CSFs resembled lung-derived CSF in functional activity, but initial estimates of molecular weights for the CSFs from the different organs ranged from 200,000 to 23,000. This puzzling apparent existence of multiple forms of CSF proved on analysis to be somewhat spurious: the estimates of molecular weight were distorted by the presence in relatively unpurified material of interacting proteins, and some of the differences in molecular weight were ascribable to a differing content of carbohydrate in the CSF as produced by different tissues.

These accumulated data made it very unlikely that a single species of CSF existed. The conclusion could no longer be avoided that the use of granulocyte-macrophage cultures had led to the detection of at least two quite different CSFs, both candidates as regulators of granulocyte-macrophage populations.

Furthermore, a more careful analysis of the CSF in post-endotoxin mouse serum and the use of antisera prepared against L-cell-derived CSF demonstrated the existence of yet another form of CSF, characterized by its curious ability only to stimulate the formation by mouse cells of minute granulocytic colonies. Purification studies, again using lung-conditioned medium, demonstrated that the granulocytic CSF was a distinct glycoprotein of molecular weight 25,000 with physical properties quite different from the other forms, particularly in its extremely high hydrophobicity.

By the late 1970s culture techniques had been developed allowing the growth of eosinophil, megakaryocyte, erythroid, and multipotential colonies, the active material eliciting these colonies being medium conditioned by lectin- or antigen-stimulated T-lymphocytes. The same medium also stimulated mast cell proliferation and was able to support some proliferation of stem cells. The natural assumption was that T-lymphocyte-conditioned medium might contain a multiplicity of biologically active molecules and possibly specific regulatory molecules for each of the cell types just listed. This was subsequently proved to be correct in part. Nevertheless, as purification work proceeded, the surprising fact slowly became evident that a single molecular form of CSF from this source material was able to stimulate the proliferation not only of granulocytic and macrophage cells, but also of eosinophils, erythroid, megakaryocytic, mast, and stem cells. The actual purification of this molecule was achieved first by the use of a simpler starting material—medium conditioned by the WEHI-3B myelomonocytic leukemic cell line—but when this CSF was finally purified from medium conditioned by normal T-lymphocytes, the molecule proved to be essentially identical.

This decade of separative protein chemistry led to the characterization by the early 1980s of four distinct types of CSF in the mouse, as summarized in Table 1. In the Hall Institute, the various CSFs are

Table 1. Biochemical nature of the CSFs

Type of CSF	Alternative names	Purified from medium conditioned by:	Molecular weight[a]	Form
Murine				
GM-CSF	MGI-IGM	Lung	21,000–23,000	Monomer
G-CSF	MGI-IG	Lung	25,000	Monomer
M-CSF	CSF-1, MGI-IM	L-cells	45,000–90,000	Dimer
Multi-CSF	IL-3	T-lymphocytes, WEHI-3B leukemic cells	20,000–28,000	Monomer
Human				
GM-CSF	Pluripoietin α, CSF α	Mo leukemia cells	14,000–35,000	Monomer
G-CSF	Pluripoietin, CSF β	5637 bladder cancer cells	18,000–22,000	Monomer
M-CSF	CSF-1	Urine, MiaPaCa pancreas cancer cells	45,000–90,000	Dimer
Multi-CSF	IL-3	T-lymphocytes	14,000–28,000	Monomer

a. Variations in apparent molecular weights of native CSFs are due to glycosylation differences.

identified by a prefix indicating the major target cell stimulated by low concentrations of the CSF. Because of the more limited human sources of CSF and the intrinsically less satisfactory human granulocyte-macrophage culture system, progress in purifying corresponding human CSFs lagged behind, but so far at least three of the corresponding human CSFs have been purified to homogeneity from tumor cell–conditioned medium. The pattern of species cross-reactivity was not uniform. Murine G-CSF and human G-CSF were active in both species; human and murine GM-CSF had no species cross-reactivity; and human M-CSF, while active in stimulating macrophage colony formation by mouse cells, had curiously minimal direct proliferative effects on human cells. A human analogue of murine Multi-CSF has now been characterized and is inactive on murine cells.

Because of the initial incorrect assumptions concerning the CSFs, it would be unwise to assume that the four types listed here are the only CSFs active on granulocyte-macrophage populations; it may well be that other types have yet to be discovered. Nevertheless, it must be emphasized that the CSFs are not simply molecules able to stimulate granulocyte-macrophage proliferation; they are the *only* known agents. For all of the very wide range of crude starting materials with stimulating activity used by various investigators, once the CSF was removed, no activity remained in the residual material.

Biochemistry of the CSFs

Certain general comments can be made regarding the properties of the CSFs as determined from the purified native molecules. First, all are glycoproteins within the somewhat broad molecular weight range of 18,000 to 90,000. Because of technical limitations, the carbohydrate content of the molecules could not be established from the small amounts of native material able to be purified from natural sources, but it can now be deduced from the known size of the recombinant polypeptides. The data indicate that carbohydrate forms approximately one-third to one-half of the weight of the various CSFs. The carbohydrate content appears to be quite variable even in CSF produced by a single cell source and differs between CSFs produced by different tissues.

Studies in which carbohydrate was stripped enzymatically from CSF, on CSF produced in nonglycosylated form by tunicamycin-treated cells, and on nonglycosylated recombinant CSFs produced by bacteria agree in indicating that the carbohydrate neither is involved in receptor binding nor influences any of the biological effects of the molecules on responding cells in vitro. Although it is possible that the carbohydrate content may influence serum half-lives or organ localization of the CSFs, it remains largely unclear why the carbohydrate is present on the molecules and whether any functional significance can be attached to the observation that different tissues appear to add differing levels of carbohydrate to the polypeptides. The variable carbohydrate content may be largely responsible for the apparent heterogeneity of different CSFs in various physical separative procedures, for example, charge-based separations.

Studies on purified native CSFs indicated that three are monomers: GM-CSF, G-CSF, and Multi-CSF. However, M-CSF, both of murine and human origin, differs in being a dimer of two apparently identical polypeptide subunits, the isolated subunits themselves having no functional activity. Further evidence for the necessity of a three-dimensional configuration of the molecules was obtained for the monomeric CSFs with the observation that mercaptoethanol was able to destroy the biological activity of all three CSFs. This predicted the existence of mandatory disulfide bridges in these CSFs, a prediction that has been confirmed by sequencing studies indicating the presence of paired cysteine residues and the construction of biologically inactive serine-cysteine muteins. Extensive studies using a variety of peptidases or cyanogen bromide to generate CSF fragments have failed to produce evidence that any small fragment of the CSFs retains detectable biological activity.

Analysis of the specific biological activity of the purified CSFs indicated that each exerts demonstrable biological activity in vitro at very low molar concentrations in the 10^{-10} to 10^{-13} M range. This information suggested that specific high-affinity receptors were likely to exist on responding cells, and this has been extensively confirmed.

From the known specific activity of the purified CSFs, it can be calculated that serum and urine CSF levels are very low (possibly in the 10–100 pg per milliliter range). Furthermore, from estimations of the recoveries of CSFs during the fractionation procedures used to purify CSF from tissue sources, the levels of CSF contained in, or released by, even the richest tissue sources are also low. For example, 10^9 mouse lungs would be required to generate 2 g of purified G-CSF.

From a consideration of the physical properties of the purified CSFs, they appear to be typical enough of an expanding group of specifically acting biological macromolecules, most of which are proving to be glycoproteins in the 10,000–100,000 molecular weight range. While the body clearly uses a variety of molecules for tissue-to-tissue signaling purposes, the use of medium-sized glycoproteins is emerging as a favored method, although the distinctive advantages of such molecules are not yet apparent.

The heterogeneity of the four known CSFs purified from native sources was somewhat puzzling since all four exhibited a variety of common functional effects on responding granulocytes and macrophages. While the CSFs might have been unrelated molecules and certainly appeared to be antigenically distinct, in the absence of detailed amino acid sequence data it remained possible that they were in fact related and were derivatives of some common ancestral regulatory molecule.

Molecular Biology of the CSFs

The entry of molecular biology into the CSF field has had a dramatic effect on progress in characterizing these molecules, not only because it allowed the complete amino acid sequence of the polypeptides to be deduced and information to be gathered regarding the organization of the CSF genes, but also because it solved the crippling logistical problem alluded to earlier, that there was simply no reasonable prospect of ever purifying enough native CSF for studies on CSF action in vivo.

For those working in the field, there had always been a latent fear that by some unverifiable misfortune the CSFs were *not* products of mammalian cells but of microorganisms that were contaminating all of the tissue sources used. At the very least, the demonstration of CSF genes in the mammalian genome has come as a great relief in eliminating this possibility.

Although molecular biology is a powerful tool, it should be noted that so far this technology has been most effective where a biological system already exists to detect the action of the molecular product of the cDNA isolated. This situation may well change, however, with the increasing use of transgenic mice to establish information on the function of an unknown gene product. In the case of the hemopoietic regulators, adequate bioassay systems existed, and studies moved ahead quickly based on the use of either semisolid cultures or highly sensitive cell lines with a known dependency for survival and/or proliferation on some type of CSF.

In principle, the isolation of the cDNA clone can be achieved either by using specific nucleotide probes synthesized on the basis of amino acid sequence data derived from the purified native protein, or by constructing cDNA libraries from some predetermined suitable cellular source and screening the library by direct expression. Both approaches were used in the isolation of cDNA clones for the different CSFs.

In view of the difficulties experienced by groups working on the purification of Multi-CSF (IL-3)—up to a 1×10^6-fold purification was required, and it was difficult to verify that the diverse actions of this molecule were indeed ascribable to a single molecular species—it was perhaps fitting that the first CSF cDNA to be cloned late in 1983 was for Multi-CSF. The two groups achieving this cloning both used direct expression screening of cDNA libraries.

Cloning of the remaining CSF genes in most cases involved the more formal route of screening cDNA libraries using oligonucleotide probes based on known amino acid sequence data from purified native proteins. Table 2 lists the various CSFs and the structure and location of their genes.

Sequencing of the CSF cDNA clones revealed a significant level of homology between corresponding human and murine CSFs. This approximated 30 to 80 percent for the nucleotides in the protein coding region. Figure 12 shows the sequences of murine and human GM-

Table 2. Molecular biology of the CSFs

Type of CSF	Deduced molecular weight of polypeptide	Exons in gene	Chromosomal location
Murine			
GM-CSF	14,000	4	11
G-CSF	19,000	5	11
M-CSF	?	?	?
Multi-CSF	15,000	5	11
Human			
GM-CSF	14,000–15,000	4	5
G-CSF	18,800	5	17
M-CSF	26,000 × 2	≥9	5
	16,000 × 2		
Multi-CSF	14,000–15,000	5	5

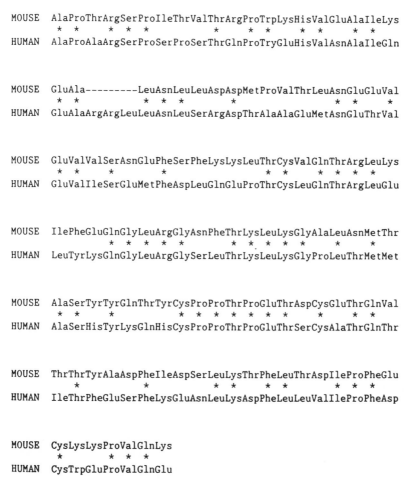

MOUSE AlaProThrArgSerProIleThrValThrArgProTrpLysHisValGluAlaIleLys
       * *   * * *   *   * *   * *   * *
HUMAN AlaProAlaArgSerProSerProSerThrGlnProTryGluHisValAsnAlaIleGln

MOUSE GluAla---------LeuAsnLeuLeuAspAspMetProValThrLeuAsnGluGluVal
       * *   * * *   *   * *   *
HUMAN GluAlaArgArgLeuLeuAsnLeuSerArgAspThrAlaAlaGluMetAsnGluThrVal

MOUSE GluValValSerAsnGluPheSerPheLysLysLeuThrCysValGlnThrArgLeuLys
       * *   *   *   * *   * * * *
HUMAN GluValIleSerGluMetPheAspLeuGlnGluProThrCysLeuGlnThrArgLeuGlu

MOUSE IlePheGluGlnGlyLeuArgGlyAsnPheThrLysLeuLysGlyAlaLeuAsnMetThr
          * * * * *   * * .* * *   *   *
HUMAN LeuTyrLysGlnGlyLeuArgGlySerLeuThrLysLeuLysGlyProLeuThrMetMet

MOUSE AlaSerTyrTyrGlnThrTyrCysProProThrProGluThrAspCysGluThrGlnVal
       * *   *   * * * * * * *   *   * *
HUMAN AlaSerHisTyrLysGlnHisCysProProThrProGluThrSerCysAlaThrGlnThr

MOUSE ThrThrTyrAlaAspPheIleAspSerLeuLysThrPheLeuThrAspIleProPheGlu
       *   *   * *   * *   * * *
HUMAN IleThrPheGluSerPheLysGluAsnLeuLysAspPheLeuLeuValIleProPheAsp

MOUSE CysLysLysProValGlnLys
       *   * * *
HUMAN CysTrpGluProValGlnGlu

Figure 12. Comparison of the amino acid sequence of murine and human GM-CSF as deduced from cDNA clones. Despite substantial homology, these CSFs do not exhibit cross-species biological activity. Note the conservation of the four cysteine residues.

CSF as fairly representative examples of the correspondence between the murine and human molecules and of the general structure of the CSFs. As predicted from mercaptoethanol studies, four cysteine residues are present linked in two bridges (1–3, 2–4), both of which are necessary for biological activity. With the use of an automated peptide synthesizer, the complete polypeptides for murine Multi-CSF and human GM-CSF have been synthesized. In agreement with previous data from the peptidase digestion of the native CSFs, major portions of the CSF molecule appear to be required for biological activity.

The sequences of all four CSFs showed no significant homology with those of any known growth factor, oncogene product, or mammalian protein, confirming earlier studies that no agents other than CSFs are capable of stimulating granulocyte-macrophage proliferation by direct action.

The most surprising information emerging from deduction of the complete amino acid sequence of each of the CSFs was that no significant homology existed between the four types; nor was there any similarity in the hydrophobicity profiles or likely secondary structure. This was clear evidence that although the CSFs share many common functions on granulocyte-macrophage populations, they are in fact quite unrelated molecules not derived evolutionarily from any conceivable common ancestral gene.

Despite this individuality of the four CSFs at the protein level, information on the genomic structure and location of the CSF genes has raised the possibility that some coordination of these genes may exist.

The genes at least for GM-CSF, G-CSF, and Multi-CSF exist in single copy form, with no closely homologous genes. Each consists of multiple exons, and for two genes (murine GM-CSF and Multi-CSF) certain cDNA clones isolated suggest that alternate splicing may be possible using an alternative first exon.

The genes for murine GM-CSF and Multi-CSF were both identified as residing on chromosome 11. Furthermore, gene mapping studies using an interspecies backcross between Mus-musculus and Mus-spretus have established that these two genes are exceedingly close together, within 250 Kbp of each other. Furthermore, a common decanucleotide that is a candidate as an initiator sequence lies 5' to the genes for GM-CSF, Multi-CSF, γ-interferon, and IL-2. These observations are intriguing because T-lymphocytes, when stimulated by mitogens or receptor antisera, exhibited a coordinated, if not entirely synchronous, major increase in the transcription of these genes with the synthesis of large amounts of secreted protein products.

An equally intriguing situation has been demonstrated in regard to the location of CSF genes in the human genome. The genes for human GM-CSF, Multi-CSF, M-CSF, and the M-CSF receptor (*c-fms*) also lie close together on chromosome 5 near the breakpoint in the 5q⁻ syndrome, a syndrome associated with a clonal proliferative disorder of granulocytic and macrophage cells. It is unlikely that this close physical association of CSF genes is ascribable to chance; the data suggest some type of genetic design in which coordinated transcription is intended.

The CSFs cannot properly be described as a "family" of regulatory molecules because of their disparate polypeptide structure. Nonetheless, at the genomic level coordination seems possible, and it exists also at the receptor level in responding cells. This is an intriguing situation whose full implications and purpose remain to be established, but it seems clear that, in referring to the CSFs, the term "functional group" is a better generic description.

The availability of cloned probes for the CSFs has allowed some studies on the capacity of various cells to alter their rates of transcription of the various mRNAs. Some cells appear able to produce additional CSF after exposure to appropriate stimuli. For various cells, the time lag to maximum secretion varies from 15 to 48 hours. Analysis of the tumor cell line Krebs II stimulated by endotoxin indicated that cytoplasmic mRNA levels for both GM-CSF and G-CSF were detectable within 1 to 2 hours and peaked at 8 hours. With T-lymphocyte cell lines, stimulated either by concanavalin A or antireceptor sera, cytoplasmic levels of mRNA for GM-CSF were already detectable after 2 hours and peaked at 12 hours. Levels of mRNA for Multi-CSF showed a similar but slightly delayed time course. In the T-lymphocyte model, the absolute elevation of CSF mRNA was at least 100-fold above basal levels.

These observations indicate that cells have the ability to alter their rates of transcription and translation of CSF very rapidly and that the alteration can be of very large magnitude, leading to the conclusion that the production of these regulators is designed to be highly labile.

Membrane Receptors for the CSFs

The lack of homology or structural similarity between the four CSFs, their glycoprotein nature, and their ability to act at very low molar concentrations predict that specific membrane receptors for the CSFs should exist and should be unique for each of the different types.

Several points of general interest emerged from studies on CSF receptors: (1) specific non-cross-reacting receptors exist for each CSF; (2) receptor numbers are relatively low; (3) receptors are restricted to cell types shown to be biologically responsive to the CSFs; (4) receptors are not restricted to cells capable of division; (5) individual cells simultaneously express receptors for more than one CSF; and (6) receptors for different CSFs functionally interact with each other.

Table 3 lists the properties of the CSF receptors on murine marrow cells. From their different sizes it is clear that the receptors are likely to be distinct molecules, and since each appears to be a monomer, the receptors cannot be composed of dimers or trimers including common subunits. The receptors for M-CSF and G-CSF are likely to be of large enough size to have intracytoplasmic domains with tyrosine kinase activity and might thus resemble in principle the well-characterized receptors for several growth factors. Indeed, studies on the M-CSF receptor have shown an ability of this receptor to undergo autophosphorylation following binding of M-CSF.

The size of the M-CSF receptor (molecular weight 165,000) and its predominant distribution on macrophage populations raised the possibility that it might be related to the c-fms proto-oncogene product of similar size and cellular distribution. Studies have shown that antisera to the c-fms product specifically bind to the M-CSF receptor, and it seems firmly established that the M-CSF receptor is either the c-fms product or is very closely related structurally. In view of the success of this approach and the general likelihood that other growth factor receptors might be related to proto-oncogene products, it seems worthwhile extending this type of correlative study.

For three of the CSFs, the average frequency of receptors on normal marrow cells appears to be quite low—in the range of a few hundred receptors per cell. However, autoradiography of marrow populations that have bound ^{125}I-labeled CSF (Figure 13) indicates that average

Table 3.   Membrane receptors for the CSFs on murine cells

Type of CSF	Molecular weight	Approximate Kd 37° C (pM)	Biological activity of CSF 37° (pM)	Range of receptor numbers on positive marrow cells
GM-CSF	51,000	20–1,000	15	70–350
	130,000			
G-CSF	150,000	100–300	3	50–500
M-CSF	165,000	30	10	1,500–10,000
Multi-CSF	75,000	100–1,000	7	50–1,000

Source: Data modified from N. A. Nicola, Immunology Today 8:134–140, 1987, table 2.

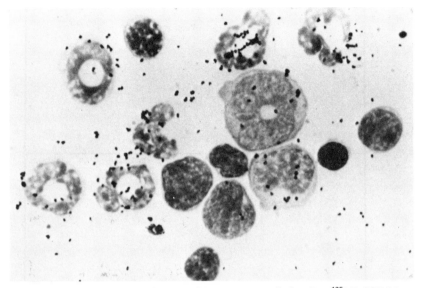

Figure 13. Autoradiograph of murine bone marrow cells binding ^{125}I G-CSF. Note that labeling is restricted to granulocytic and monocytic populations and that postmitotic polymorphs exhibit the highest level of binding.

binding data do not give a very accurate picture of actual receptor numbers on individual cells. Some cells in the marrow such as nucleated erythroid cells or B-lymphocytes possess no receptors, and since these two populations total at least one-quarter to one-third of the total marrow population, actual receptor numbers on binding cells are correspondingly higher. Furthermore, receptor numbers differ widely within any one lineage according to differentiation state. In the example shown in Figure 14 of G-CSF labeling of murine marrow cells, it is evident that the most mature cells in the granulocytic lineage, the polymorphs, exhibit considerably higher receptor numbers than do less differentiated cells in the series. It is also evident that within any one subpopulation, up to 50-fold heterogeneity exists in the number of receptors, making it hard to express average receptor numbers even for cells of one subclass.

The basis for the heterogeneity exhibited by cells of a single subclass has not been established. Cell cycle–based differences cannot account for the variability, since extensive variability is also exhibited by postmitotic polymorphs. More likely explanations are (1) that receptor numbers expressed at any one time may reflect the immediate past history of the cell; if it had recently made contact with G-CSF or

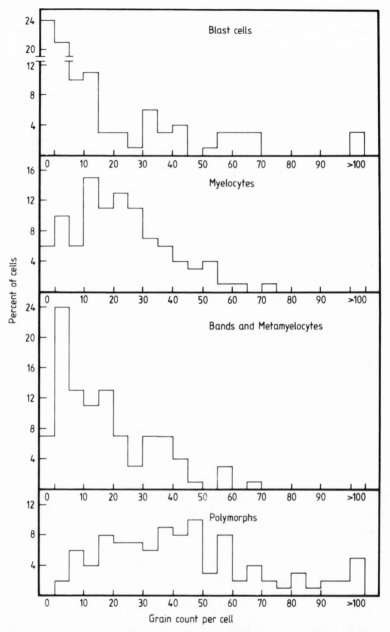

Figure 14. Histograms of grain counts from autoradiographs of murine bone mar-row cells labeled with [125]I G-CSF. Note the heterogeneity of labeling of individual cells within any one differentiation class, and that postmitotic polymorphs exhibit the highest overall levels of labeling.

another CSF in vivo, G-CSF receptors might be temporarily down-regulated; or (2) that receptor numbers may reflect some more general physiological state of the particular cell, including its age or state of functional activation.

In the case of marrow blast populations, subsets exist that lack receptors for each of the CSFs. Here a more obvious explanation is possible, namely that some blast cells are in unrelated lineages such as the erythroid or lymphoid. This would merely be an extension of the observation that the more differentiated members of these sub-populations also clearly lack receptors for the CSFs. A similar conclusion can be drawn from a consideration of the labeling pattern of purified progenitor cells, a subpopulation of cells identified as blast cells and again a mixed population committed to different cell lineages. These purified progenitor populations also exhibit obvious positive and negative subsets, and so, for example, it can be presumed that some erythroid progenitors do not exhibit CSF receptors.

This permits an interesting deduction concerning the nature of the differentiation process occurring during progenitor cell commitment. As will be discussed in Chapter 4, both Multi-CSF and to a lesser degree GM-CSF have proliferative actions on at least some stem cells and on multipotential and early erythroid progenitors. Although it has not been possible to purify such populations selectively and examine directly whether or not they display CSF receptors, logic suggests that at least some must express such receptors. It seems possible, therefore, that differentiation commitment of such cells to become more mature erythroid progenitor cells must be accompanied by cessation of expression of CSF receptors on the membrane of these cells. It has been possible in the past to postulate two alternative models of receptor expression during differentiation (Figure 15). In the first model, stem cells display no specific regulator receptors, and entry of cells into a committed state is based on an acquired capacity to synthesize and display the necessary lineage-related receptors. In the second model, stem cells can be visualized as displaying a wide range of lineage-restricted receptors. In this model, entry of a cell into the committed progenitor cell stage is based on selective suppression of expression of irrelevant receptors.

The exact CSF receptor status of purified mouse stem cells should be able to be established from autoradiographic studies on these cells. Once such a study has been performed, it should be possible to decide which of these two models of differentiation commitment is correct.

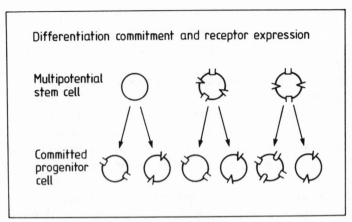

Figure 15. Three methods by which multipotential stem cells might generate committed progenitor cells: *(left)* commitment might involve the expression of membrane receptors for appropriate regulatory molecules; *(center)* stem cells might express receptors for all possible regulators and commitment might involve cessation of expression of inappropriate receptors; *(right)* the commitment process might involve both suppression of preexisting receptors and the display of new types of receptors.

From the data available on morphologically identifiable cells, there are no examples of display of CSF receptors by a more differentiated cell where less mature cells in the lineage do not display such receptors. However, it is also clear that there is no constant pattern of decreasing or increasing receptor expression with increasing differentiation. Thus while G-CSF receptor numbers on murine cells increase with increasing differentiation, receptor numbers for the same molecule on human cells show an opposite pattern in which promyelocytes exhibit the highest receptor numbers. A similar lack of consistent pattern is seen when one analyzes receptor numbers for the other CSFs.

In the case of Multi-CSF and M-CSF, a further complexity exists in that, for both, a small subset of marrow cells exhibits extraordinarily large numbers of receptors, outside the wide range of variability already described. For Multi-CSF, the situation is quite puzzling because these highly labeled cells exhibit no constant morphology, some being blast cells while others have a quite differentiated morphology resembling myelocytes or metamyelocytes. In view of the wide spectrum of cell types responding to Multi-CSF, it is possible that these cells bearing ultra-high receptor numbers are members of a distinct hemopoietic sublineage.

It has been possible to establish a number of cloned continuous hemopoietic cell lines from murine cells that are of uncertain differentiation lineage and are abnormal in regard to various features such as their capacity for self-generation and their karyotype. These will be discussed later in the context of leukemogenesis, but it is of interest to note here that these highly responsive cell lines are absolutely dependent on Multi-CSF for survival and proliferation. They have also been shown to display exceptionally high average numbers of receptors for Multi-CSF (10,000 to 50,000 per cell). One obvious question raised by these cell lines is whether they are derived from the rare cells in normal marrow expressing similarly high receptor numbers.

Another question raised by these highly responsive cell lines is whether the absolute number of receptors on a cell correlates with, or determines, its responsiveness to stimulation by a particular CSF. Individual granulocyte-macrophage progenitors are highly heterogeneous in their responsiveness to stimulation by CSF, and conceivably this also parallels the variation in receptor numbers on these cells. Because antireceptor antisera are not now available, it is not yet technically possible to sort progenitor cells and test the relative CSF-responsiveness of cells with high versus low receptor numbers. However, this type of study is technically possible with T-lymphocytes, and it has been demonstrated that cells exhibiting the highest numbers of IL-2 receptors are also the most highly responsive to proliferative stimulation by IL-2. This type of correlation seems likely also to apply to CSF responsiveness and may be one basis for the observed heterogeneity of progenitor cells to stimulation by CSF.

One earlier hypothesis concerning the nature of the postmitotic state in a differentiating cell system was that this was a consequence of cessation of expression of membrane receptors for the relevant growth factor. However, the presence of membrane receptors for the CSFs on postmitotic polymorphs excludes this as a mechanism responsible for the postmitotic state, at least for cells in the granulocytic lineage.

Comparison of the percentage of cells binding each of the four murine CSFs indicates that most granulocytes and monocytes at all differentiation stages from the progenitor stage onward must simultaneously express receptors for at least three and possibly all four CSFs (Table 4). If the CSFs indeed represent the main regulators of granulocyte-macrophage populations, their similar actions indicate a high level of redundancy in the design of the control system. The advantages served by such a design are not yet clear, but the presence of

Table 4.   Binding of iodinated CSFs to murine bone marrow cells

Cell type	Mean grain counts (% positive)			
	G-CSF	GM-CSF	Multi-CSF	M-CSF[a]
Blast cells	19 (76)	80 (90)	60 (88)	+
Promyelocytes/myelocytes	24 (94)	90 (100)	66 (100)	+/−
Metamyelocytes	16 (85)	60 (100)	34 (95)	+/−
Polymorphs	44 (100)	64 (100)	26 (100)	+/−
Promonocytes	8 (77)	94 (100)	63 (100)	+
Monocytes	4 (57)	48 (100)	36 (96)	+ +
Eosinophils	0	29 (93)	61 (100)	0
Lymphocytes	0	0	0	0
Nucleated erythroid cells	0	0	0	0

Source: Data modified from N. A. Nicola, *Immunology Today* 8:134–140, 1987, table 3.

a. Grain count data not available for M-CSF. Level of binding indicated as follows: 0 = none; +/− = low levels of binding; + = binding; + + = high levels of binding.

multiple CSF receptors on each individual cell appears to provide the physical basis for receptor-receptor interactions and the competitive and enhancing effects seen when hemopoietic populations are exposed to combinations of CSFs.

The relatively low numbers of CSF receptors on hemopoietic cells suggest that individual receptors could be widely separated on the membrane, and no evidence suggesting receptor clustering has been observed in any autoradiographic analysis. Despite these data, a very interesting situation has been observed regarding concentration-dependent interactions between receptors for the different CSFs. In competition binding studies performed at 0° C, there is no evidence that any CSF can bind to the receptors for the other CSFs. However, if such studies are performed at 37° C, occupation by one CSF of its receptors can be shown to result in significant down modulation of other types of CSF receptors. This down-modulation tends to be unidirectional and to fall into a hierarchical sequence, as shown in Figure 16. Thus occupation by Multi-CSF of its receptors on marrow cells leads to a reduction in the ability of all three remaining types of CSF receptor to bind to their respective ligands. Prebinding of the other three CSFs does not influence the capacity of the Multi-CSF receptors to bind Multi-CSF. Similarly, binding of GM-CSF to its receptors down-modulates G-CSF and M-CSF receptors. The evidence is less

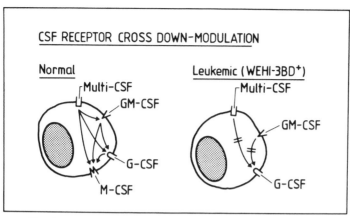

Figure 16. The hierarchy of CSF receptor down-modulation on normal murine marrow cells. In WEHI-3B D$^+$ myeloid leukemic cells this down-modulation sequence is disrupted, and binding of either Multi-CSF or GM-CSF fails to down-modulate G-CSF receptors.

clear on the relative hierarchical positions of G-CSF and M-CSF receptors, but the data slightly favor the conclusion that G-CSF receptors tend to be the dominant member of the pair.

The mechanisms responsible for this down-modulation are unknown but are likely to involve induced cytoplasmic cascades, since physical proximity of the receptors is unlikely. However, it is not known whether the other CSF receptors remain in place in the membrane, whether selective conformational changes occur in the receptors, or whether some generalized membrane change is involved that alters the display of other receptors on the membrane including those for the CSFs. The last possibility seems unlikely in view of the unidirectional nature of the down-modulation phenomenon. Also unknown is whether the net consequences of down-modulation result in inactivation of the receptor involved or in a state of functional activation.

As expected from the ability of low concentrations of CSF to exert detectable biological effects, the receptors have proved to have high binding affinities. Binding kinetics of the CSFs to their receptors at 0° C are very rapid and are essentially irreversible. For most CSFs the ligand-bound receptor complex becomes protease-insensitive, although for some, binding can be reversed by lowering the pH. Internalization of the ligand-receptor complex is rapid for M-CSF ($t\frac{1}{2}$ of a few minutes) but somewhat slower for Multi-CSF ($t\frac{1}{2}$ 15–60 minutes).

Similarly, the rate of breakdown of internalized bound receptor complexes varies with the different CSFs and also with the type of cell involved. For example, breakdown of M-CSF-receptor complexes is extremely rapid in peritoneal macrophages but much slower in marrow-derived macrophages, while the breakdown of internalized Multi-CSF-receptor complexes is relatively slow ($t\frac{1}{2}$ 2–3 hours). In general, the rate of reexpression of membrane CSF receptors is relatively slow ($t\frac{1}{2}$ 1–6 hours), meaning that, for cells exposed to CSF, a major fraction of all CSF receptors are in fact intracytoplasmic in location at any one point in time (75 percent in the case of Multi-CSF receptors under equilibrium conditions).

Some evidence has been presented that cells do not need to be exposed to CSF continuously for CSF-induced effects to be detectable. However, the slow turnover of bound CSF receptors in many situations seems likely to permit sustained intracellular signaling from bound receptor complexes. This makes it difficult to determine by direct observation whether episodic stimulation by CSF can act merely as a trigger initiating a self-sustaining series of metabolic cascades, or whether continuous signaling is required to sustain even the briefest type of detectable response.

The curious binding and internalization characteristics of the CSFs make it difficult to establish true equilibrium binding constants by conventional Scatchard analyses. However, the equilibrium dissociation constants (Kd) appear in general to be higher than the concentrations of CSF required to elicit half-maximal proliferative responses, suggesting that such responses may be achieved with low levels of receptor occupancy despite the relatively small numbers of available receptors on many cells.

Although exposure of cells to CSF has been found to result in changes in the rate of synthesis of many cytoplasmic and nuclear proteins and in their phosphorylation, the observed changes are too complex to allow any comment on the detailed cytoplasmic events following the binding of a CSF to its receptors.

Summary

The four colony-stimulating factors thus far identified in the mouse and man controlling the proliferation of granulocyte-macrophage populations have all been purified, and cDNAs for each have been cloned. All are glycoproteins, three being monomers and one a dimer, and they do not share sequence homology. Unique membrane receptors exist for each CSF, but most granulocyte-macrophage cells simultaneously express receptors for several, possibly all, CSFs. The dissimilar nature of the four CSFs is curious in view of their similar biological effects and raises obvious problems to be resolved concerning the purpose and advantages of what appears to be an unnecessarily redundant control system. Despite their dissimilar nature, patterns of intended coordinated action of the CSFs are beginning to emerge both from a consideration of the structure and location of the CSF genes and from evidence of interactions between different CSF receptors on individual responding cells.

4

Biological Effects of the CSFs on Hemopoietic Cells In Vitro

The granulocyte-macrophage CSFs were originally detected and later purified on the basis of the mandatory role they play in stimulating the proliferation of precursor cells in this population. As this work proceeded and purified CSFs became available for further investigation, it became apparent that these molecules were not simply proliferative stimuli. Indeed, they are now known to have a variety of direct actions on cells on responding populations, which can be summarized as follows: (1) enhancement of cell survival in vitro, (2) stimulation of cell proliferation, (3) differentiation commitment, and (4) enhancement of functional activity of mature cells.

This combination of functional properties seemed highly unusual at the time but in fact is now emerging as a typical pattern for more recently characterized hemopoietic regulators and for regulators of nonhemopoietic tissues. It has perhaps been simpler to recognize the variety of actions possessed by the CSFs because of the availability of high-efficiency culture systems for the *primary* culture of unaltered hemopoietic cells—techniques not yet available for most cell types—and because granulocyte-macrophage populations exhibit functions that are well characterized and readily measured.

Enhancement of Cell Survival In Vitro

The initial observations on enhancement of cell survival showed that if CSF was initially withheld from cultures of hemopoietic cells and then added after a progressive delay, a progressive reduction was observed in the number of colonies developing (Figure 17). The conclusion was that the CSFs were necessary for the survival and/or

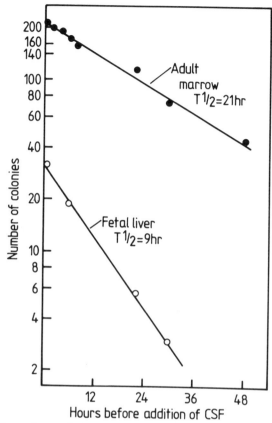

Figure 17. Failure of granulocyte-macrophage progenitor cells from adult mouse marrow or fetal liver to survive in cultures initiated without CSF. When GM-CSF was added after varying intervals, progressively fewer colonies resulted.

retention of proliferative capacity of progenitor cells in vitro. More careful sequential analysis of such cultures showed that in fact the progenitor cells died in the absence of CSF.

Although the effects of CSF withdrawal on clonogenic progenitor cells or continuous cell lines are spectacular and readily reproducible, it seemed unlikely that similar effects would be observable with mature granulocytes or monocytes because these populations had been studied in vitro for years under conditions likely to have been CSF-free. However, recent studies on mature human polymorphs and eosinophils have demonstrated that addition of CSF can significantly enhance in vitro survival, and this phenomenon is demonstrable using CSF concentrations below those necessary to stimulate cell proliferation.

Some evidence has been produced to indicate that the actions of the CSFs in maintaining cell viability in vitro are due to their ability to maintain intracellular ATP levels and an intact membrane glucose transport system.

Withdrawal of M-CSF from M-CSF-dependent cultures of marrow-derived macrophages led to a 100-fold fall in DNA synthesis, a decreased rate of protein synthesis, and a rise in the rate of protein degradation. These effects may be the consequence of failure to maintain membrane integrity or may represent additional metabolic abnormalities induced by CSF withdrawal that lead to premature cell death.

It is unclear whether the CSFs might have similar actions on responding cells in normal in vivo conditions. However, when Multi-CSF-dependent mast cell lines were injected subcutaneously, surviving cells could only be demonstrated in animals injected with Multi-CSF-containing material; thus a possibility exists that CSFs can exhibit this function in vivo. With the availability of recombinant CSF, it would be of interest to determine whether the injection of CSF can increase the life span of mature granulocytes and monocytes in vivo.

Stimulation of Granulocyte-Macrophage Proliferation

The ability of the granulocyte-macrophage CSFs to stimulate precursors of these cells to proliferate and form colonies of maturing progeny was the basic property that allowed the CSFs to be discovered and characterized, and colony stimulation remains the hallmark for categorization of a particular macromolecule as being a member of the CSF group. It might be wondered whether this functional classification is not a piece of circular logic that carries with it the real risk of generating a quite artificial "group," since the molecules are quite different and only share in common the property of being proliferative stimuli.

The validation of this functional grouping has come from evidence of associated transcription of the molecules, interactions between specific CSF receptors, the ability of one CSF to alter production rates of another, and evidence of common intracytoplasmic signaling pathways initiated by the CSFs. This more recent evidence has retrospectively validated what was at first little more than an operational convenience—the categorization of the CSFs as a functional group.

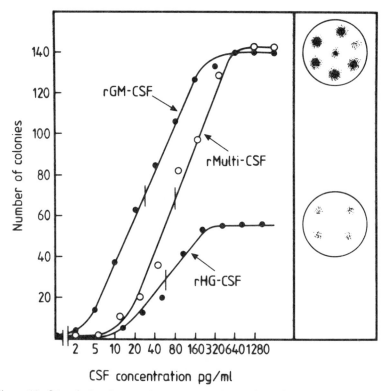

Figure 18. Stimulation by varying concentrations of purified recombinant GM-CSF, Multi-CSF, or G-CSF of granulocyte-macrophage colony formation by progenitor cells from mouse bone marrow. Note that G-CSF stimulates the formation of relatively few colonies, all of which are small in size.

The increasing evidence for interactions between the CSFs makes their apparently unique role as mandatory stimuli for cell division in granulocyte-macrophage populations all the more remarkable. No other purified growth factor is capable of initiating proliferation in these populations. No metabolic enhancement of the medium results in proliferation, and the few agents able to stimulate proliferation in vitro, such as the phorbol esters, do so indirectly by provoking the production and/or release of CSF by other associated cells.

A characteristic dose-response curve is observable in semisolid cultures between the concentration of CSF used and the number of colonies developing (Figure 18). A number of features of this dose-response curve are worthy of comment. The CSFs are able to exert their proliferative effects at extremely low concentrations in the 10^{-10} to 10^{-12} range. It is also evident that the different CSFs, when at supramaximal concentrations, stimulate differing absolute numbers of colonies to develop. These differences are paralleled by differences in the proportion of granulocytic, granulocyte-macrophage, and macrophage colonies (Table 5). Thus in cultures of mouse bone marrow cells, M-CSF stimulates the formation predominantly of macrophage colonies, and only a low frequency of granulocytic or granulocyte-macrophage colonies develops even with very high M-CSF concentrations. GM-CSF stimulates the formation of similar absolute numbers of colonies, but these are of all three types. At low concentrations only macrophage colonies develop, but as GM-CSF concentrations are elevated, up to 60–70 percent of the developing colonies contain or are composed entirely of granulocytic cells.

In terms of granulocyte-macrophage colony formation, Multi-CSF behaves like GM-CSF although without the preponderance of macrophage colonies at low concentrations. G-CSF exhibits characteristic differences. The total number of colonies that develop following stimulation by G-CSF is never more than 30–40 percent of the number that develop with the other CSFs. Furthermore, after 7 days of incubation, the colonies are of very small size, most colonies being composed of pure populations of unusually mature granulocytic cells. Only with quite high G-CSF concentrations do low numbers of granulocyte-macrophage or macrophage colonies develop, and these never reach the number or size of those developing with M-CSF or GM-CSF.

The fact that a sigmoid dose-response relationship exists between CSF concentration and the number of colonies developing indicates

Table 5. Frequency of various colony types formed by murine bone marrow cells stimulated by 50 units per milliliter of the different CSFs

Type of CSF	Mean number of colonies	Percentage of colonies				
		G	GM	M	Eo	Disp
GM-CSF	65	20	10	70	0	0
G-CSF	14	91	9	0	0	0
M-CSF	45	3	15	82	0	0
Multi-CSF	55	19	17	32	2	30

Note: For work with the stimulation of colony formation by CSFs, 50 units is defined as the concentration in a 1-ml culture stimulating the formation of half-maximal numbers of colonies. G = granulocyte, GM = granulocyte-macrophage, M = macrophage, Eo = eosinophil, Disp = dispersed natural cytotoxic.

that different progenitor cells are heterogeneous in their quantitative responsiveness to stimulation by CSF; some are able to proliferate when exposed to low concentrations while others require concentrations that are 10 to 100 times higher before they can proliferate.

These differences in responses to different CSFs and CSF concentrations form the basis for the conclusion alluded to earlier that granulocyte-macrophage progenitor cells are a quite heterogeneous population of clonogenic cells. That this heterogeneity is real and not simply the result of stochastic processes aborting the extent or duration of responsiveness of a particular clone is demonstrated by the ability of cell separation procedures to segregate, albeit incompletely, subsets of progenitor cells with different proliferative patterns following stimulation. By these procedures, highly responsive cells can be separated by size from less responsive cells, and cells generating granulocytic colonies can be segregated by density or FACS fractionation from those generating granulocyte-macrophage or macrophage colonies.

Colonies are somewhat arbitrarily defined as clones containing more than 40 to 50 cells after an incubation period, usually of 7 days. In any culture of marrow cells stimulated by a CSF, there is also present a larger group of smaller clones of varying sizes—the so-called granulocyte-macrophage clusters. Physical separative procedures have been quite successful in segregating cluster-forming from colony-forming cells, again indicating that stochastic processes do not abort colony-forming cell proliferation merely to lead to cluster formation. The two clonogenic populations are genuinely different although linked in a parent-progeny relationship, cluster-forming cells being the immediate progeny of colony-forming cells.

Much of the heterogeneity evident in a CSF-stimulated culture can reasonably be ascribed to the occurrence of a heterogeneous series of commitment events in the stem cell compartment during the generation of the progenitor cells. There are certain aspects of the heterogeneity that remain puzzling, however, and G-CSF-stimulated colony formation is an outstanding example of the problems still to be resolved. The absolute numbers of granulocytic colonies stimulated to develop by G-CSF approximately equal the absolute numbers of granulocytic colonies developing in cultures stimulated by GM-CSF or Multi-CSF, but the G-CSF-stimulated colonies differ in being smaller and more differentiated. The simplest explanation of these differences is to postulate that identical granulocyte progenitors are involved but that some action of G-CSF leads to accelerated maturation to postmitotic cells, aborting further expansion of the colony. This would predict that mixing of G-CSF with GM-CSF or Multi-CSF would result in some acceleration of maturation of granulocytic colony cells, with size reduction in developing granulocytic colonies. In fact, the opposite is observed: in cultures containing both G-CSF and GM-CSF, maturation of granulocytic colony cells is not accelerated, and the resulting colonies are larger than with GM-CSF alone. It could be speculated that macrophage or granulocyte-macrophage progenitors might lack receptors for G-CSF, thus accounting for the failure of G-CSF to stimulate the formation of these types of colonies. However, autoradiographic data from binding of G-CSF strongly suggest that this is not the case and that macrophage and granulocyte-macrophage precursors do exhibit G-CSF receptors. A more compelling experiment is to observe the early events in G-CSF-stimulated colony formation and to determine what happens when a G-CSF-initiated clone is transferred to a culture containing GM-CSF or Multi-CSF. What is observed is that G-CSF initiates the proliferation of far more clones than ultimately survive and form colonies. After 2 to 4 days of incubation most G-CSF-initiated clones stop proliferating, die, and disintegrate. When 2- to 3-day-old G-CSF-initiated clones are transferred to cultures of GM-CSF or Multi-CSF, most continue proliferation and form granulocyte-macrophage or macrophage colonies. Conversely, most clones initiated by GM-CSF or Multi-CSF die after transfer to G-CSF-containing cultures, and the small number surviving generate typical small granulocytic colonies.

This evidence suggests that G-CSF initiates the proliferation of the same subset of granulocyte macrophage progenitor cells as GM-CSF or Multi-CSF but that, as the clonal progeny begin to differentiate, G-CSF is unable to stimulate their further proliferation. This interpretation is supported by the inability of G-CSF to act as a functional stimulus for mature macrophages, but because the mixing experiments argue against accelerated maturation, it does not explain the small size of granulocyte colonies that do develop with G-CSF. Furthermore, G-CSF receptors are present on all maturing granulocytic and monocytic cells, and therefore loss of responsiveness due to intracolony maturation cannot be ascribed simply to loss of G-CSF receptors. Combination of the above data leads to the conclusion that the apparently simple phenomenon of small granulocytic colony formation following stimulation by G-CSF cannot be explained on the basis of what is known at present concerning CSF actions. To a degree, this admission of failure probably applies to other colony types regarding the causes of their distinctive heterogeneity in composition and size.

The clone transfer technique has proved to be a versatile and revealing method for analyzing hemopoietic colonies developing in semisolid cultures. If the procedure is performed with care, intact clones can be transferred with little or no surrounding agar medium, and any CSF carried over is rapidly diluted beyond effective concentrations by diffusion into the recipient agar cultures. A refinement of this technique is the transfer of individual washed cells from such clones. Use of both techniques has shown that CSF must be present throughout the culture period if clonal proliferation is to be maintained. Most clones transferred to CSF-free cultures immediately stop proliferation and die within 1 to 2 days. Developing murine macrophage colony cells are particularly susceptible to CSF withdrawal, and when single cells are transferred to CSF-free cultures, they invariably fail to complete any further divisions and die within 24 hours. Developing murine granulocytic colony cells can be more resistant in the absence of CSF, one-third can complete one or two further divisions before dying. Human granulocyte-macrophage colony cells are somewhat slower to exhibit the effects of CSF withdrawal, but much the same phenomena ultimately occur.

Some evidence has been produced to suggest that the CSFs may need to operate only during the G_1 phase of the cell cycle. However, this seems improbable in view of the failure of cells from most Multi-CSF-dependent cell lines to complete a single division following withdrawal of Multi-CSF. Furthermore, according to the CSF and cell type involved, prolonged persistence intracellularly of CSF-receptor complexes is possible that would result in sustained intracellular signaling throughout a typical cell cycle of 8 to 15 hours' duration. Even if further evidence confirms that CSF is not necessary during late events in the cell cycle, all data agree that the CSFs are not simply initiating triggers that are able to achieve within minutes all that is necessary for a cell to proceed from G_1 to completion of cell division.

One of the characteristic features of CSF-stimulated colony formation by normal or responsive neoplastic cells is that the mean size achieved within a defined time interval increases with increasing CSF concentrations. This observation suggests strongly that the CSFs may exert a concentration-dependent influence on mean cell cycle times. This is an important issue because an initial criticism of the CSF studies was that the CSFs may simply be molecules that prevent cell death in vitro and, by so doing, permit the cells to remain healthy and to exhibit an intrinsic capacity for cell proliferation that is not at all dependent on extrinsic signaling. Given that the CSFs are indeed necessary for cell survival, this criticism is pertinent and must be answered.

There are two major problems that prevent simple deductions from being made from the familiar influence of CSF concentration on colony size. First, developing granulocyte-macrophage colonies after the first few days contain differentiating cells many of which may no longer be capable of further division. If CSF can somehow delay maturation to postmitotic cells, this action alone would be sufficient to allow colonies to achieve a larger size. The argument is less valid for colonies grown from CSF-dependent cell lines, where again there is a clear relationship between CSF concentration and colony size because most colony cells do not mature and remain clonogenic.

The second problem is that both normal and neoplastic granulocyte-macrophage clonogenic cells are clearly heterogeneous in response to stimulation by CSF. If this heterogeneity were associated with intrinsic differences in proliferative potential, it could lead to misinterpretation of the observed correlation between CSF concentration and colony size. Such an association has indeed been observed with granulocyte-macrophage progenitor cells from mouse bone marrow. Velocity sedimentation separation studies (segregating cells according to size) have shown the existence of distinct subsets of progenitor cells: (1) cells forming small macrophage colonies that respond to very low CSF concentrations; (2) cells forming large granulocyte-macrophage colonies that are less responsive to stimulation; and (3) cells that require a very high CSF concentration to proliferate but then generate large multicentric granulocytic colonies.

These two problems required elaborate studies to provide definitive evidence that the CSF concentration *does* influence cell cycle times. The studies used paired daughter cells of normal or continuous cell line clonogenic cells separated by micromanipulation; the cells were then washed and subsequently cultured in parallel in cultures with different CSF concentrations. Clone size increase was monitored at intervals by direct visual counting during the subsequent 48 hours' incubation. A requirement of the analysis was that, with both concentrations, increase in clone size should be logarithmic during the observation period to eliminate possible differentiation-based suppression of certain cells of the clone.

With both cell populations used, evidence was obtained that higher CSF concentrations shortened average doubling times (mean cell cy-

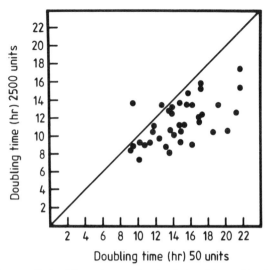

Figure 19. Mean cell doubling times of paired daughter cells of granulocyte-macrophage progenitor cells grown in different concentrations of GM-CSF. Doubling times are shorter for the daughter cell stimulated by the higher GM-CSF concentration than for the matching daughter cell stimulated by the lower GM-CSF concentration.

cle times; see Figure 19). This property of the CSFs seems therefore to have been established, but the cellular mechanisms responsible remain unknown.

The same studies also showed that the final colony size achieved after 7 days of incubation was also larger with daughter cells grown in the higher CSF concentration. Shortened cell cycle times could account for the observed size difference, but since normal colony populations ultimately contain differentiating and postmitotic cells, the increased size of normal colonies might possibly have been due to the fact that high CSF concentrations tended to delay maturation. This latter question has been analyzed using colonies grown from continuous cell lines, but CSF concentration was found not to influence the proportion of clonogenic cells in a colony.

Lineage-Specificity of Proliferative Actions of the CSFs

The four CSFs were initially found to be proliferative stimuli for granulocyte-macrophage cells except in the case of Multi-CSF, where it was evident, once the CSF had been purified to homogeneity, that

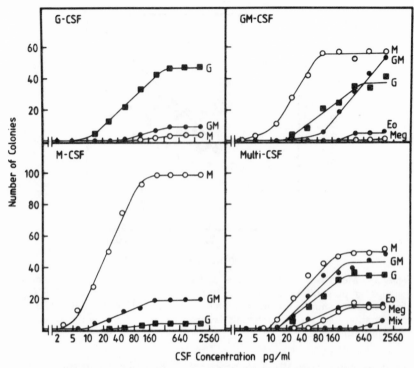

Figure 20. Effects of increasing the concentration of purified CSF on the number of colonies of different types developing in cultures of murine bone marrow cells. G = granulocytic; GM = granulocyte-macrophage; M = macrophage; Eo = eosinophil; Meg = megakaryocytic colonies.

this CSF had proliferative effects on a much broader range of hemopoietic cells. At first this seemed to set Multi-CSF apart from the other three types, but with the availability of adequate amounts of purified native and recombinant CSFs it has become clear that, when CSF concentrations are increased, there is a progressive broadening in the action of all three of these CSFs, perhaps best shown by GM-CSF (Figure 20).

At concentrations below 20 pg per milliliter, GM-CSF is a proliferative stimulus only for macrophage colonies. In the concentration range 20–40 pg per milliliter, GM-CSF becomes a proliferative stimulus for apparently all available macrophage, granulocyte-macrophage, and granulocyte progenitor cells. Above 80 pg per milliliter GM-CSF becomes an effective proliferative stimulus for eosinophil progenitors, and above 640 pg per milliliter an equally effective stimulus for all available megakaryocyte progenitors and for at least some multipotential progenitors. At no concentration yet tested does GM-CSF stimulate the proliferation of mast cells. A more limited version of this phenomenon is seen with both M-CSF and G-CSF, although the proliferative actions are restricted to cells of the granulocyte-macrophage differentiation lineage.

A very similar range of cross-linear actions can be documented by initiating cell proliferation with one CSF and then adding a second, more appropriate one. This sequential addition technique can employ lower CSF concentrations than are needed in studies using a single CSF. Thus the fact that low concentrations of GM-CSF have direct, if temporary, proliferative effects on some multipotential and erythroid precursors can be demonstrated by initiating cultures using GM-CSF and then on day 2 adding Multi-CSF to sustain and complete the formation of pure and mixed erythroid colonies. Since the same result can be achieved using cultures of a single erythroid or multipotential progenitor cell which can be observed to divide up to five times before the Multi-CSF is added, the phenomenon is a clear demonstration of direct cross-reactivity.

G-CSF can be shown to have the same action on multipotential and erythroid progenitors, but the proportion of such cells responding is lower and little evidence of initial proliferation can be observed in culture mapping studies. M-CSF appears to have no action on multipotential cells in this type of sequential addition experiment.

Because GM-CSF has early proliferative effects on some murine BFU-E and erythropoietin has proliferative effects on murine CFU-E (the progeny of BFU-E) but not on BFU-E themselves, it should be possible to grow some BFU-E-derived erythroid colonies using a combination of GM-CSF and erythropoietin, and this has indeed been observed.

The mechanisms responsible for the broadening of action of a molecule like GM-CSF as concentrations are increased are unclear. All of the cell populations responding to high GM-CSF concentrations do exhibit receptors for GM-CSF, confirming that the cross-lineage actions are direct. One obvious possibility is that a cell will be stimulated to proliferate only if more than the minimum absolute number of receptors is occupied. This would not only be a reasonable explanation of the differing quantitative responsiveness of various granulocyte-macrophage progenitors but would also account for cross-lineage actions at high CSF concentrations if, for example, multipotential, erythroid, or megakaryocytic progenitors have only a small number of CSF receptors. Since cross-lineage proliferation can be initiated with lower GM-CSF concentrations than are required for colony formation when GM-CSF alone is used, it is possible that initiation can occur with fewer occupied receptors than are required for sustained proliferative stimulation. Alternatively, maturing cells of other lineages in a colony may express fewer GM-CSF receptors than do progenitor cells or their initial progeny. This latter explanation seems more probable for cells in the erythroid lineage, since recognizable erythroid cells express no GM-CSF receptors.

Binding competition studies and autoradiography indicate that GM-CSF cannot occupy Multi-CSF receptors and cannot down-regulate these receptors. Therefore, the effects of the sequential use of GM-CSF followed by Multi-CSF cannot be ascribed simply to activation by the GM-CSF of Multi-CSF receptors.

No evidence has been obtained for the existence of specific CSF receptors on T- and B-lymphocytes, fibroblasts, or other nonhemopoietic cells. This is paralleled by the failure to demonstrate direct effects of the CSFs on any of these cell types. The possibility of indirect effects will be discussed in Chapter 7.

The CSFs and Granulocyte-Macrophage Maturation

A major issue raised by the ability of the CSFs to stimulate the formation of maturing cells of other lineages is the question of whether the CSFs directly regulate cellular maturation as well as proliferation. The cells in normal colonies stimulated by the CSFs exhibit progressive maturation as incubation proceeds (Figure 21). Since similar maturation occurs in cultures using serum-free fully defined culture medium and in cultures initiated with the use of a single cell, there is a strong temptation to conclude that the CSFs do control maturation, for example the progression of cells from myeloblasts to polymorphs.

Maturation by hemopoietic cells is likely to require the sequential activation of a large number of cellular genes. For example, in granulocyte maturation, these genes would need to encode changes in nuclear morphology, the sequential formation of primary and then secondary granules, the synthesis of a variety of specialized end cell macromolecules, and the acquisition of phagocytic and killing mechanisms. In theory, these multigene changes could well be linked into a single, sequentially self-activating, transcriptional sequence. It is obvious, however, that a differentiation program for neutrophilic gran-

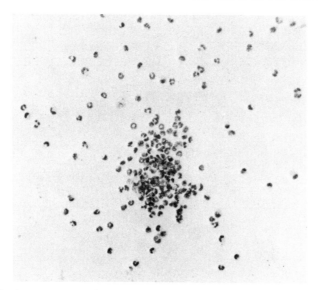

Figure 21. A murine granulocytic colony stimulated to develop by G-CSF. Such colonies are noted for their small size and their uniform content of mature cells.

ulocytes would need to be quite different from that for macrophages or eosinophils.

The question at issue here is whether GM-CSF is likely to be able to activate all three types of differentiation program and whether one can therefore describe it as "controlling" maturation. It is conceivable that GM-CSF-receptor signaling could induce a single transcriptional event whose product would be capable of initiating a self-sustaining transcription cascade for either neutrophil, monocyte, or eosinophil maturation. The actual transcriptional cascade triggered would be dependent on prior genetic programing occurring during lineage commitment of the cell. With this arrangement, GM-CSF would be able to initiate the eventual formation of typical mature polymorphs, monocytes, or eosinophils (Figure 22). In a certain sense, this could be described as "controlling" maturation. However, the usual usage of a word like "controlling" implies a much more intimate and continuing role in a process, with an ability to regulate by direct intervention some or all of the sequential maturation events. It seems very improbable that a single CSF-initiated signal could possibly regulate in detail the very large number of transcriptional and translational events required in the formation of a mature cell in any lineage, let alone in three different lineages. Furthermore, some mechanism

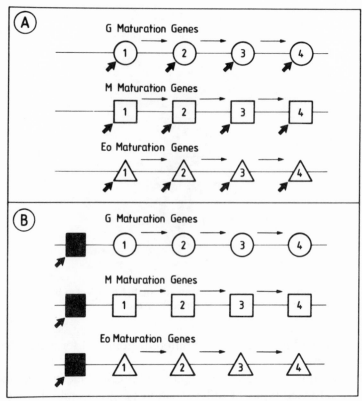

Figure 22. Schematic representation of the multiple genes necessary for pro-graming maturation changes in granulocytes (G), macrophages (M), and eosinophils (Eo). Ordered activation of transcription of these genes is probably required to produce a mature cell. The sequential activation could be maintained by autostimulation, and the genes need not be on the same chromosome. It is improbable, as in part A, that CSF-initiated products could directly alter the transcription of each of these multiple genes. However, it may be possible, as in part B, that a CSF-initiated product could activate a signaling region common to all three gene groups and initiate a series of autostimulating transcriptional events. Which actual sequence was activated would depend on preprograming occurring during lineage commitment.

would be required to prevent bizarre aberrations of maturation in which, for example, eosinophil granules would develop in poly-morphs.

To justify the use of an expression such as "control," it would also be necessary to show that differing concentrations of a CSF could influence the transition time of, for example, a myelocyte to a metamyelocyte, or the rate of nuclear morphological changes associated with polymorph maturation. No such studies have been reported.

A number of experiments indicate that "inappropriate" ligand-receptor signaling can initiate proliferative responses similar to those initiated by the binding of the "correct" ligand to its receptors. Thus transfection of mRNA for the M-CSF receptor to fibroblasts with subsequent expression of M-CSF receptors on the cell membrane leads to an ability of M-CSF to stimulate fibroblast proliferation, and similar experiments using IL-2 receptor transfection to uniquely Multi-CSF-responsive cell lines led to the cells becoming responsive to IL-2. It is clear, therefore, that the initial events following the formation of ligand-receptor complexes must be common for a number of these complexes. However, for the reasons discussed earlier, the consequences of such initial signaling are more likely to be determined by which differentiation program sequences are available for activation in the cell involved. Thus the activatable state of a particular differentiation program sequence is the crucial commitment event that will result eventually in the occurrence of a particular maturation sequence.

The CSFs appear to be able to influence the activatable state of a particular differentiation program, and it is in this restricted context that CSFs can perhaps be described as "influencing" maturation. However, this influence relates only to the choice of pathway initiated rather than to any capacity to modulate subsequent events in detail. Future experiments may indicate that this view underestimates the ability of the CSFs to influence cellular maturation, but the question is intrinsically difficult to investigate because the CSFs are necessary for cell survival and no simple comparison is possible of maturation of healthy cells in the presence and absence of CSF.

Induction of Differentiation Commitment by the CSFs

In Chapter 1 evidence was discussed indicating that major differentiation restriction events in multipotential hemopoietic stem cells seem to be stochastic in nature, because no predictable pattern has been observed in the manner in which oligopotential or monopotential cells are generated following cell division. It was emphasized, however, that all random events occur with a certain probability, and that this probability need not be constant or incapable of alteration by extrinsic signaling.

Bipotential granulocyte-macrophage progenitors, particularly in the adult mouse, offer a simple model system for analyzing a restricted type of differentiation commitment involving the exclusive formation of granulocytic or macrophage progeny. In cultures of mouse granulocyte-macrophage progenitor cells stimulated by GM-CSF or Multi-CSF, approximately equal numbers of granulocyte, granulocyte-macrophage, and macrophage colonies develop. An early indication that these colony ratios might not be fixed was the demonstration that when highly purified progenitor cells were stimulated by either M-CSF or GM-CSF, most cells formed colonies. However, in the M-CSF cultures the large majority of colonies contained only macrophages, whereas in the cultures stimulated by GM-CSF a high proportion of the colonies contained granulocytes. This observation suggested that the type of CSF used might have some ability to influence which type of progeny develops in at least some of the colonies.

This observation was extended by growing colonies from micromanipulated paired daughter cells, with one daughter cell cultured in a high GM-CSF concentration and the other in a low GM-CSF concentration. In this study, some progenitor cells appeared already to be unipotential and to generate only granulocytic or macrophage progeny regardless of the concentration of CSF used. However, for about one-third of the daughter cell pairs, GM-CSF concentration did influence the type of progeny developing, with granulocytic progeny appearing only in cultures containing high GM-CSF concentrations (Figure 23)—a result that helps to explain the known dose-response effects of GM-CSF referred to earlier.

Both types of observation were criticized on the ground that the results were possibly due to selective survival—granulocytic cells simply being unable to survive in cultures with low GM-CSF concentrations. This type of criticism was rendered less tenable by studies in which clones were initiated either by GM-CSF or M-CSF and then transferred to cultures containing the same or the alternate CSF. Similar crossover studies were also performed using washed individual daughter or granddaughter cells. All three types of experiment showed that initiation of cell proliferation by M-CSF tended to lead to macrophage colony formation when clones or cells were transferred subsequently to cultures containing GM-CSF. Conversely, GM-CSF-initiated clones or cells remained capable of generating some granulocyte-containing colonies when subsequently stimulated in cultures containing M-CSF. This procedure, which resulted in large, healthy

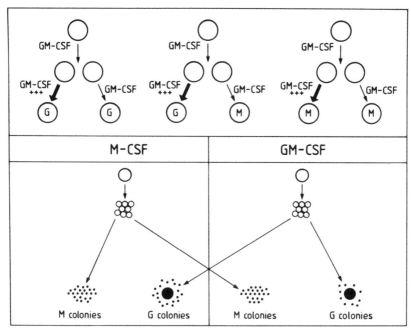

Figure 23. Two examples of differentiation commitment by CSFs. In the upper panel, daughters of one-third of bipotential cells *(center)* generate granulocyte-containing colonies in cultures containing high GM-CSF concentrations, while the paired daughter cells generate macrophage colonies in low GM-CSF concentrations. In the lower panel, clones initiated by M-CSF form exclusively macrophage colonies when transferred to GM-CSF-containing cultures; clones initiated by GM-CSF continue to generate some granulocyte-containing colonies after transfer to cultures containing M-CSF.

granulocytic colonies developing in cultures containing M-CSF, was quite impressive when contrasted with the uniform macrophage nature of colonies in cultures stimulated from the outset by M-CSF. The phenomenon was more evident with day 2 and day 3 clones containing 8 to 16 cells than after the transfer of single daughter cells, and it was more evident with granddaughter cells than with daughter cells. This suggests that cells need to pass through one or several cell divisions before commitment by the CSF in use becomes irreversible.

This commitment phenomenon can be explained by postulating that binding of M-CSF to its receptors is able to initiate events leading to irreversible shutdown of the potential granulocyte differentiation program existing in a bipotential cell, and thus that the CSFs are able to influence differentiation commitment to the degree of being able to shut off a potential differentiation program. It must be pointed out, however, that there are examples of CSF-stimulated cell division where no commitment appears to occur. The most striking example is the ability of GM-CSF to stimulate up to five divisions in erythroid precursors without altering the subsequent exclusive formation of erythroid progeny by these cells. This suggests that the ability to alter potential differentiation programs could be significantly limited, perhaps by the nature and programing of the responding cells.

The ability of the CSFs to irreversibly influence differentiation programs in responding bipotential granulocyte-macrophage progenitor cells would predict that the combined use of two different CSFs should lead to competitive commitment and the formation of mixed granulocyte-macrophage colonies. This has in fact been observed in cultures containing M-CSF combined with either GM-CSF or G-CSF. With both combinations, the proportion of mixed colonies is higher than with either stimulus alone (Table 6). In typical granulocyte-macrophage colonies, the granulocytic component tends to be central and to be surrounded by presumably more motile macrophages. However, in the mixed colonies resulting from the use of two CSFs, often the granulocytic focus is strikingly eccentric. The strong implication is that at least one of the early progeny of the bipotential cell is committed irreversibly to granulocyte formation in competition with the macrophage-committing action of the M-CSF.

A further example of the ability of CSFs to irreversibly alter the program of cells leading to differentiation commitment will be discussed in Chapter 10 in reviewing the action of G-CSF in inducing

Table 6.   Enhancement of colony stimulation by combination of CSFs

Stimulus	Mean number of cells per colony	Mean absolute number of colonies per culture		
		Granulocytic	Granulocyte-Macrophage	Macrophage
M-CSF	160 ± 95	0	1	44
GM-CSF	101 ± 132	6	6	17
G-CSF	120 ± 100	7	2	2
M-CSF + GM-CSF	317 ± 160	2	22	30
M-CSF + G-CSF	370 ± 220	7	18	43

Note: Cultures contained 25,000 C57BL bone marrow cells and M-CSF 330 units, GM-CSF 40 units, or G-CSF 100 units alone or in combination. Colonies in four replicate cultures were analyzed after 7 days of incubation.

commitment of leukemic cells to enter terminal differentiation. Again, the process requires passage of the cells through one to two cell divisions in the presence of G-CSF and is irreversible and asymmetrical in nature.

Although the examples of differentiation commitment are limited, they do provide evidence that extrinsic signaling can irreversibly influence choices made by responding cells by either activating or suppressing possible differentiation programs. It is in this context that the CSFs can be regarded as having some influence on maturation in hemopoietic cells, albeit by influencing only an early step in such maturation sequences.

Stimulation by CSFs of the Functional Activity of Mature Granulocyte and Macrophage Cells

Although it has long been recognized that some classical hormones can influence multiple parameters in responding tissues, including both growth stimulation and functional activities, most of these studies were performed in vivo, where there was no good evidence that a particular response was necessarily due to direct action of the molecules. Indeed, general thinking two decades ago envisaged separate molecules as controlling cell proliferation and the functional activity of mature cells, since the necessary cellular events were likely to be quite different and possibly antagonistic.

Work with hemopoietic regulators and particularly the CSFs has now shown that stimulation of proliferation and of end cell functional activity can be controlled by the direct actions of the same molecules.

A variety of direct actions of purified CSFs have now been documented on purified populations of mature polymorphs, monocyte-macrophages, and eosinophils (Figure 24). There are certain common characteristics associated with these responses:

1. Most responses are rapid and become measurable within minutes or hours of exposing the cells to the CSF.

2. The responses probably require the continuous presence of the CSF, since levels of cell activity return to normal after withdrawal of the CSF.

3. The concentrations of CSF required to elicit functional responses are no higher than those required to elicit proliferation of precursor cells, and in some cases can be considerably lower.

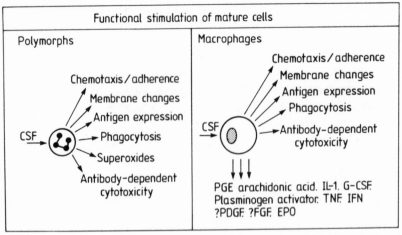

Figure 24. Functions of mature granulocytes and monocytes able to be stimulated by the direct action of appropriate CSFs.

4. The same lineage specificities of the CSFs observed for proliferative responses are also observed with functional activation. Thus GM-CSF but not G-CSF can stimulate eosinophil function, while both GM-CSF and G-CSF can stimulate neutrophil function.

5. Responses are initiated by the direct action of the CSFs on the responding mature cells, but the actual response observed may be due to production by the responding cells of another biologically active molecule—the regulator cascade phenomenon.

A minimum requirement for establishing a *direct* action of CSFs on mature end cells is to perform the test in vitro using purified target cells, a requirement that rules out certain types of studies such as adherence to endothelial cells, penetration of endothelial layers, or release of cells from the marrow. Cellular events of the latter type can only be monitored in vivo, where certification of direct CSF action is not possible, and thus it is likely that the list of observed functional effects of the CSFs on mature cells is quite incomplete. Few in vitro functional tests have been performed on single cells or under limiting dilution conditions where the nature of the response could be determined. Thus the responses listed below are certainly *initiated* by direct CSF action, but whether the end effects are sometimes mediated by other secreted molecules remains an open question.

Observed responses of human and/or murine cells to CSF include the following:

1. GM-CSF is chemotactic for both polymorphs and monocytes. When cells are located at the position of highest GM-CSF concentration, their motility is inhibited. GM-CSF is the factor described previously as neutrophil migration inhibitory factor (NIF).

2. The CSFs affect the shape of polymorphs, monocytes, and eosinophils, at high concentrations often elongating the cells and causing an irregular margin possibly due to membrane ruffling. They also influence the rate of uptake of glucose and Na^+K^+-ATPase-mediated uptake of rubidium.

3. GM-CSF and G-CSF increase the phagocytic activity of polymorphs and their ability to kill ingested microorganisms. GM-CSF and M-CSF also exert similar actions on monocytes and macrophages.

4. GM-CSF increases autofluorescence of eosinophils and increases superoxide production in neutrophils.

5. GM-CSF and G-CSF stimulate increased antibody-dependent cytotoxicity of polymorphs for tumor cells. GM-CSF and Multi-CSF stimulate eosinophil cytotoxicity in a similar assay, while M-CSF stimulates increased cytotoxicity of macrophages for tumor cells; the latter action is indirect, through the induced production of tumor necrosis factor.

6. GM-CSF stimulates increased RNA synthesis in polymorphs and the increased synthesis of a number of unidentified nuclear and cytoplasmic proteins.

7. The CSFs have been observed to stimulate the formation by monocytes of interferon, tumor necrosis factor, prostaglandin E, arachidonic acid, interleukin-1, and plasminogen activator.

8. M-CSF and Multi-CSF are able to stimulate murine macrophages to produce G-CSF; human GM-CSF stimulates human monocytes to produce M-CSF, and human M-CSF stimulates human monocytes to produce a granulocyte-stimulating factor, probably G-CSF. GM-CSF has been observed to stimulate murine erythroid cell proliferation if macrophages are present, possibly by stimulating the production of erythropoietin by macrophages.

9. The CSFs stimulate increased membrane expression of certain antigens characteristic of mature granulocytes and monocytes.

The behavior of CSF-stimulated cells in vitro is similar to the observed behavior of neutrophils, macrophages, and eosinophils at sites of inflammation. Thus the CSFs seem likely to be members of the group of mediator molecules responsible for attracting cells to an inflammatory site and then activating them to increased metabolism and functional activity. Although the CSFs are unique as the only known direct proliferative stimuli for granulocyte and macrophage precursors, they are unlikely to be the only agents stimulating functional activity of mature end cells.

Summary

Analysis of the actions of the CSFs on responding hemopoietic cells in vitro has demonstrated that these molecules exhibit a broad series of effects ranging from proliferative stimulation to functional activation. The ability of cells to respond and the nature of the actual response occurring depend on two types of genetic programing in the cells: (1) that leading to the synthesis and display of specific receptors for the CSFs, and (2) that determining whether the cells proliferate, enter defined differentiation pathways, or exhibit enhanced functional activity. Thus the genetic programing of the target cells is the dominant factor determining their responses to the CSFs, although the equation is not wholly one-sided because the CSFs do have a subtle capacity to alter this programing during differentiation commitment responses.

At least for M-CSF and G-CSF, the evidence indicates the existence of only one type of membrane receptor; thus the diverse effects of the CSFs are initiated by the common event of binding of the CSF to this single membrane receptor class (Figure 25). Activation of the receptor, possibly by phosphorylation, must be presumed to be able to initiate a multiplicity of secondary metabolic cascades, many of which are likely to result in membrane or cytoplasmic effects. Some, however, must be capable of transmitting information to the nucleus, since cell division and differentiation commitment require signals to enter the nucleus and perhaps impinge on quite selected regions of various chromosomes.

Although the three-dimensional configuration of the CSFs could allow these molecules to contain information able to initiate some metabolic cascades, current concepts favor the view that ligands serve

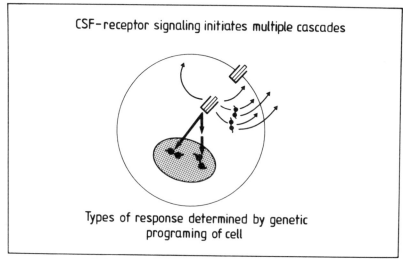

Figure 25. Representation of three types of responses able to be initiated by the binding of a CSF to its membrane receptor. The multiple metabolic cascades occurring following binding can induce (1) local changes in the membrane, (2) the synthesis of various proteins, or (3) irreversible changes in gene programing. Which type of response is most prominent appears to be determined by the genetic preprograming of the responding cells.

only to activate receptors, and that it is the activated receptor alone that initiates all subsequent responses. The data on this question do not seem unequivocal at present. The number of ligand molecules must equal the number of activated receptors, and where there is no gross disparity in molecular size or complexity, as is true for some CSF-receptor pairs, it is not immediately obvious why the receptor, rather than the ligand, is the only possible activating molecule. If the receptor should be closely linked structurally to molecules mediating subsequent events, this would of course make the receptor more likely to be the active molecule. In this context, the large size differences between various CSF receptors are puzzling because the types of responses elicited by the CSFs are in general similar. The murine M-CSF receptor is capable of autophosphorylation following activation, and the G-CSF receptor is large enough to code for a similar tyrosine kinase domain. The other two murine CSF receptors seem too small to permit this phosphorylation mechanism and would need to achieve activation by some alternative mechanism.

One suggestion for circumventing this difficulty regarding the similar effects but differing receptor sizes of the CSFs has been the proposal that there are in fact two functional classes of CSF receptors: (1) those able to initiate both cell proliferation and differentiation, but with an action favoring proliferation (for Multi-CSF and GM-CSF); and (2) those concerned mainly with inducing differentiation effects (for G-CSF and M-CSF). At least in the mouse, this functional grouping also corresponds with a distinct size difference, the receptors for Multi-CSF and GM-CSF being distinctly smaller than those for G-CSF and M-CSF. In this interpretation, many of the differentiation effects of Multi-CSF and GM-CSF would be mediated by their capacity to down-modulate the receptors for G-CSF and M-CSF (assuming down-modulation in this situation to be equivalent to functional activation).

Evidence supporting this hypothesis comes from the behavior of these receptors on continuous cell lines and leukemic cells that fail to differentiate and also fail to exhibit down-modulation of G and M receptors. The suggestion here is that GM-CSF and Multi-CSF fail to induce terminal differentiation in such cells because of the functional disruption of the down-modulation sequence. As will be shown in Chapter 10, G-CSF is effective in inducing leukemic cell differentiation, perhaps by bypassing this block.

It is also of interest that the most common continuous cell lines are dependent on either Multi-CSF or GM-CSF, and that even if a line such as NFS 60 also responds to stimulation by G-CSF, G-CSF cannot sustain continued cell proliferation of this line as can the other two CSFs.

There are, however, some obvious weaknesses in this proposal as presently formulated. Continuous M-CSF-dependent cell lines do exist, and both G-CSF and M-CSF are clearly active in stimulating cell proliferation. Furthermore, GM-CSF *can* induce moderate differentiation in leukemic cells despite its failure to down-modulate G-CSF receptors on these cells. Despite these weaknesses, the hypothesis has some merit in attempting to explain the purpose of CSF receptor interactions, and further experimental analysis seems warranted.

Although it is possible to question whether receptors alone initiate the variety of cytoplasmic changes able to be elicited by the CSFs, it seems likely that neither the CSF molecules nor their receptors are the molecules that enter the nucleus to mediate the necessary nuclear changes. This is for the simple reason that so few molecules are involved that their dilution after finally entering the nucleus would not permit any likely types of chemical interaction. Further progress in determining how CSF elicits such nuclear responses will depend on identification of amplifying mediator molecules generated in the cytoplasm following binding of CSF to its receptor.

One of the most discussed questions in cell biology is whether maturation (or differentiation) can only occur in association with, or following, cell division. The reason for this controversy is that, at least in some situations, differentiation is asymmetrical, implying that the newly synthesized daughter chromatid is the one affected, and because it seems more feasible to alter gene programing irreversibly, for example by methylation, when the chromosome is in an extended form during the S-phase of the cell cycle. The available evidence from hemopoietic cells certainly favors the occurrence of asymmetry during differentiative divisions, and in the CSF-induced commitment events, cell division seems to be necessary. It is not surprising, therefore, that a mediator molecule like CSF should be able to influence both proliferation and differentiation commitment. What remains surprising is the ability of the same molecules to exert such powerful functional effects on postmitotic mature cells. This economy in the control system appears to compensate for the unnecessary redundancy of using four distinct molecules to achieve similar proliferative responses, often by identical target cells. Possible reasons for the existence of four CSFs rather than a single one are beginning to emerge from a consideration of the actions of the CSFs in vivo, to be discussed in Chapter 7.

5

Sites and Control of CSF Production and Degradation

If the mandatory role of the colony-simulating factors in stimulating granulocyte and macrophage formation in vitro is valid evidence that CSFs regulate the formation of these cells in vivo, it is of importance to establish the cellular sources of the CSFs and the nature of the mechanisms regulating their levels and rates of production.

Cellular Sources of the CSFs

In principle, four quite different sets of cells could be envisaged as being able to produce CSFs (Figure 26). First, CSF production could be restricted to cells of the hemopoietic system itself (intrinsic sources). The cells involved could either be immature or mature granulocyte-macrophage cells, or specialized microenvironmental cells within the hemopoietic tissues. Alternatively, the CSFs could be produced by nonhemopoietic cells (extrinsic sources). These could either be a set of cells widely dispersed throughout tissues dependent on the functional actions of granulocytes and macrophages, such as endothelial cells or fibroblasts, or *all* cells in the body.

For all four types of cellular sources, CSF production might either occur at a fixed rate or be capable of varying according to differing demands. Given the complexity of situations arising in both normal health and disease states, extrinsic or intrinsic sources of CSF need not be mutually exclusive alternatives, and the relative importance of each could vary according to circumstances.

Some general comments can be made concerning the suitability of extrinsic versus intrinsic cellular sources. A system relying entirely on instrinsic CSF sources has some obvious limitations. First, if granulo-

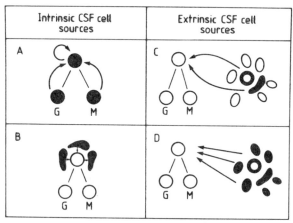

Figure 26. Possible cellular sources of the CSFs. Cells producing CSF could be within hemopoietic tissues and either be hemopoietic cells (*A*) or microenvironmental cells (*B*). Alternatively, cells producing CSF may be dispersed throughout nonhemopoietic tissues (*C*), or possibly all cells have some capacity to produce CSF (*D*).

cytes and macrophages themselves were the sole source, the situation in principle would be similar to that envisaged for some types of cancer where the cells behave in an autocrine manner, producing their own growth factors. This simple concept of cancer is inadequate to explain the behavior of a cancer cell; nevertheless, a self-stimulating cell system might be intrinsically prone to cancer development. Second, exclusive production of CSFs by granulocytes and macrophages would be unable to elicit the formation of the first granulocytes and macrophages during ontogeny and would also be unlikely to permit efficient regeneration of this population following injury. Third, CSF products exclusively formed by microenvironmental cells within the hemopoietic tissues would avoid both these problems but would not efficiently meet the needs of regeneration following local hemopoietic damage. More important, this would not be an efficient method for generating high local CSF concentrations in nonhemopoietic tissues, a desirable situation where functional activation of mature cells is required to cope with localized problems such as a focus of invading microorganisms.

Extrinsic CSF sources would suffer none of these design disadvantages in coordinating granulocyte and macrophage formation throughout the body or in responding to increased local demands for CSF but would leave unexplained why granulocyte and macrophage formation, if exclusively CSF-dependent, is localized only in the bone marrow and spleen, especially since some progenitors circulate in the peripheral blood.

From the outset of work on the CSFs, two facts emerged: (1) CSF was detectable in the serum, indicating that, at least in part, the CSFs function as humoral regulators. This eliminated the most extreme version of the intrinsic source possibility where the CSFs were displayed solely on the membranes of microenvironmental cells. (2) CSF was present in, and produced by, many nonhemopoietic tissues. This excluded hemopoietic tissues as an exclusive intrinsic CSF source and eliminated the possibility that CSFs might have a single organ source, as is the situation with classical hormones.

It has been found in the mouse that CSF is extractable from all major organs in concentrations higher than those in the serum, and studies on eight major mouse organs indicated that all were able to synthesize GM-CSF, G-CSF, and probably M-CSF. Some differences were apparent between organs, with the salivary gland, thymus, lung, and kidney having a higher content and synthetic capacity than other organs, but the differences were not large (2-fold to 6-fold). It is important to emphasize that levels of CSF extractable from marrow or spleen tissue were not outstandingly high, nor was their ability to synthesize CSF in vitro.

These findings suggested either that the CSFs might be products of all tissue cell types, or that there might be certain cells common to all tissues that are the source of the CSFs. Resolution of these two alternatives has yet to be achieved. It is usually necessary to test 10^5 to 10^6 cells per milliliter to detect CSF synthesis by bioassay, and few cell types can be obtained in pure form in such numbers.

Certain cell types are relatively easy to obtain and test. It is now known that lymphocytes, macrophages, fibroblasts, marrow stromal cells, and endothelial cells, but probably not polymorphs, can produce one or more of the four types of CSFs (Table 7). However, this positive information has had the unfortunate consequence of making it difficult to establish whether other cell types produce CSF. Thus the fact that the kidney produces CSF may be due simply to its content of vascular endothelial cells, fibroblasts, and occasional monocytes but equally might be due to the fact that all of the many cell types in the kidney produce CSF.

The functional capacity of tumors or tumor cell lines is often examined on the basis that information obtained might reveal the functional activity of corresponding normal cells. However, this is a dubi-

Table 7. Normal cells able to synthesize CSFs

Cell type	Murine	Human
T-lymphocytes	GM-CSF, Multi-CSF	GM-CSF, Multi-CSF
Monocytes	GM-CSF, G-CSF	GM-CSF, G-CSF, M-CSF
Fibroblasts	M-CSF, GM-CSF	M-CSF, GM-CSF, G-CSF
Marrow stromal cells	M-CSF, GM-CSF, G-CSF	GM-CSF, G-CSF
Endothelial cells		GM-CSF, G-CSF, M-CSF

Note: In many cases, CSF transcription and synthesis are only demonstrable following the use of inductive stimuli.

ous proposition given the chromosomal derangements common in such tumors and the possible abnormal derepression of various genes in such cells. To the extent that tumor-derived information is at all valid, the evidence suggests that a wide variety of cell types could be CSF producers because cancers of many types, such as carcinomas of various tissues, sarcomas, melanomas, and leukemias, have been found to produce CSF.

Two procedures may ultimately permit more satisfactory information to be obtained: the use of monoclonal antibodies to detect cellular CSF, and in situ hybridization to detect cellular mRNA. However, no satisfactory studies using either technique have been reported, and both techniques have significant limitations in sensitivity that could result in a serious underestimation of CSF-producing cells.

The available information thus clearly supports the conclusion that CSF production is not restricted to cells of hemopoietic tissues and that, at a minimum, CSFs are produced by a variety of cell types present in all organs. The limited knowledge of the exact cellular sources of the CSFs is emphasized by a consideration of the source materials used in the first purification of each of the murine CSFs. M-CSF was purified from L-cell conditioned medium; although these cells are fibroblasts, they have been in culture for many years and may no longer be exhibiting the exact synthetic behavior of normal fibroblasts. Multi-CSF was purified from lectin-stimulated spleen cell conditioned medium, where analysis showed that the T-lymphocyte was the active cell, a conclusion subsequently supported by work using cloned T-lymphocyte cell lines. Whether lymphocytes resident in vivo produce CSF is still undocumented. In the case of GM-CSF and G-CSF, the source used was medium conditioned by lung tissue from mice preinjected with endotoxin. It is still quite unclear which cell type or types produce the CSFs in this commonly used conditioned medium.

The situation in the fetus, at least in the mouse, seems to differ from that in adults in that M-CSF is prominent in the yolk sac, fetal liver, and blood early in fetal development and may possibly be the only CSF produced at this stage. In this context it is of interest that the uterus contains M-CSF and that M-CSF levels are increased by estrogens and rise to extremely high levels during pregnancy, again raising the possibility that M-CSF plays a dominant role in fetal hemopoiesis perhaps because of the need for extensive macrophage-mediated tissue remodeling.

Much of the work on tissue production of the CSFs was performed before the existence of multiple types of CSF was recognized, and many uncertainties remain about the relative amounts of these CSFs produced by various tissues. There is also some uncertainty about whether the circulating levels of the three CSFs reflect actual tissue production rates. Recent evidence indicates that in the adult mouse, most serum CSF may be M-CSF, with lesser amounts of G-CSF and possibly very low amounts of GM-CSF. This suggests that serum CSF levels may not passively parallel tissue CSF production but may be regulated by some more positive mechanism.

Similar uncertainty exists regarding the origin of the CSF in normal urine, which is almost exclusively M-CSF. The obvious possibility is that this CSF is cleared from the plasma by the kidney. However, kidney tissue and presumably bladder and other urinary tract tissue produce CSF, and a proportion of urinary CSF may actually be secreted into the urine by cells of the kidney and urinary tract. In general, high serum CSF levels are paralleled by high urinary CSF levels, but in GM-CSF transgenic mice with high serum GM-CSF levels (see Chapter 9), only male mice excrete GM-CSF in the urine and the concentrations are higher than those in the serum, indicating that the mechanisms by which CSF appears in the urine might be quite complex.

The most puzzling current problem regarding the location of CSF production concerns Multi-CSF. In vitro, the cell type able to produce Multi-CSF is the stimulated T-lymphocyte, with only a single report indicating Multi-CSF production by any other cell type, namely skin epithelial cells. However, Multi-CSF cannot be detected in the serum, urine, or any hemopoietic, lymphoid, or tissue extract or medium conditioned by such tissues. Similarly, no Multi-CSF mRNA has been detected in any tissue. The extraordinary situation is that Multi-CSF

has yet to be detected in the normal body, yet normal marrow populations constitutively express specific membrane receptors for this
molecule.

Regulation of Tissue CSF Production

Bioassays on serum CSF levels in various abnormal situations have
shown that they can vary over a 100-fold to 1,000-fold range. Similar
variations have been noted in production rates of CSFs by various
cells after inductive signaling. It is therefore evident that CSF production can be highly labile, and although some cells may be capable of a
constitutive synthesis of relatively constant levels of CSF, other cell
types clearly must be capable of being induced to greatly increased
rates of transcription, translation, and synthesis of CSF.

In principle, signals to vary CSF production could be products of
normal cells either of the hemopoietic cell population or of tissues
outside this population (Figure 27). Alternatively, signals could be
abnormal in nature and enter the body from the exterior. Further
possibilities are that signals act directly on CSF-producing cells or
indirectly by first interacting with other cells which then release sig-

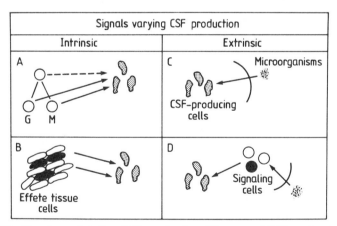

Figure 27. Signals modulating CSF production. The rate of CSF production may
be influenced by products of hemopoietic cells (A) or of hemopoietic stromal cells
(B). Alternatively, signals could arise external to the hemopoietic tissues, the most
potent being products of microorganisms (C). Signaling of the latter type might
arise indirectly and be initiated by mediator molecules released from other cell
types (D).

naling molecules activating or suppressing CSF production. The fact that multiple cell types are known to produce CSF predicts that inductive signals for increased CSF synthesis are likely to be multiple and to vary for different cell types.

Signals originating within hemopoietic or other tissues resulting in increased CSF synthesis could be of a variety of possible types: (1) decreased production of some product of mature granulocytes or macrophages; (2) increased production of breakdown products of mature granulocytes or macrophages following destruction of these populations; (3) signals from organs containing tissue or cells in need of destruction by macrophages, for example, during organ remodeling or destruction of aging cells; or (4) signals from tissue in need of repair following injury, infection, or both. The most likely type of extrinsic signal would be products of invading microorganisms and/or damaged tissue resulting from infection by such organisms.

Evidence for Intrinsic Signaling

The most effective agents for damaging hemopoietic populations are cytotoxic drugs and whole-body irradiation. If significant negative or positive signaling resulted from widespread destruction of granulocytic and macrophage populations, both types of agents should elicit pronounced increases in serum and/or tissue CSF levels. Elevation of serum CSF levels has been reported following whole-body irradiation, with levels paralleling the dose used. Similarly, drug-induced neutropenia has been observed to result in elevated serum CSF levels. However, in conventional animals, both situations are complex because there is associated gut damage, which allows the possibility of an associated endotoxemia. It is significant that serum CSF levels do not rise in germ-free animals after whole-body irradiation. More recent studies at the Hall Institute using pathogen-free mice have also failed to find significant elevations in serum CSF levels after either whole-body irradiation or cytotoxic drugs.

Serum CSF levels are high in the fetus (presumably relatively germ-free and likely to be undergoing extensive tissue remodeling) and are also high in the pregnant uterus, which is not normally subject to infection. Serum CSF levels are elevated in mice bearing many types of spontaneous, virus-induced, or transplanted tumors and in some humans with advanced cancers of various types. The mechanisms responsible for the elevated CSF levels could include some type of demand for cell destruction (that is, host resistance to tumor tissue), but in many instances the tumor tissue itself is the source of the additional CSF and the elevated circulating CSF levels are simply the consequence of unrestrained CSF synthesis by tumor cells. In other instances there is a likelihood that advanced cancer is associated with secondary infections and that the latter could be responsible for elevating CSF levels, although tumor-bearing germ-free mice also can exhibit elevated CSF levels.

The changes involved in all these situations involving tissue damage, tissue remodeling, or cancer are usually relatively small in magnitude, and although such signaling might well be sufficient to provoke low levels of CSF production, the changes are trivial in magnitude compared with those induced by extrinsic signaling.

Evidence for Extrinsic Signaling

Early evidence that extrinsic signaling was the most likely initiator of major changes in CSF production was the observation that serum CSF levels are extremely low or undetectable in germ-free and pathogen-free mice. Conversely, the injection of endotoxin in mice begins to elevate serum CSF levels within an hour. The serum CSF increases can be up to 60,000 units per milliliter (1,000-fold higher than normal levels), with peak levels being achieved between 2 and 8 hours (Figure 28). The increase is mainly due to increased levels of M-CSF and G-CSF, with only a minor rise in GM-CSF levels. Elevated CSF levels decline to normal within 24 hours of an injection of endotoxin, but repeated daily injections of endotoxin induce repeated CSF elevations until endotoxin unresponsiveness finally develops.

Similar responses can be elicited by bacterial flagellin and a variety of whole bacterial vaccines, but responses to foreign proteins are relatively weak or absent. The implication is that it is not the foreignness per se of the microbial products but their pharmacological properties that elicit the responses. Other evidence against the endotoxin-induced response being immunological in nature or lymphocyte-mediated is the fact that endotoxin produces similar responses in irradiated or athymic mice in vivo and has inducing effects in vitro on isolated vascular endothelial cells and macrophages.

Similar elevations of serum CSF levels to those induced by endotoxin are observed in the acute stages of infections in animals and man. These infections can be viral, bacterial, or protozoal in nature, but all elicit marked increases in serum CSF levels that are sustained until the fever subsides.

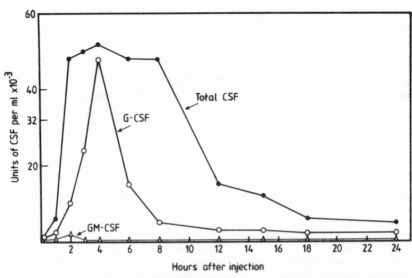

Figure 28. Increase in serum CSF levels in C57BL mice injected intravenously with 5 μg endotoxin. The increase in total CSF levels is a composite of a minor rise in GM-CSF and a major rise in G-CSF, with the remainder being M-CSF.

T-lymphocytes exhibit an extraordinary capacity to synthesize GM-CSF and often Multi-CSF in vitro following stimulation by lectins, alloantigens, or antireceptor sera. Rises in transcription of mRNA for GM-CSF precede those for Multi-CSF, become detectable within 1 to 2 hours of stimulation, and are maximal at 12 hours, with maximal levels of secreted CSF being achieved by 15 to 24 hours. During peak responses, the level of CSF synthesis is 1,000-fold above resting levels.

This type of T-lymphocyte response could in principle be activated by antigens of intrinsic origin, for example, age-related changes in red cell antigens or autoantigens in autoimmune disease. However, sera from patients with active autoimmune diseases do not show elevated CSF levels, and it is perhaps more likely that the most common antigens activating T-lymphocyte responses are of microbial origin.

Taken together, the data strongly suggest that the most potent factor inducing alterations in CSF production is signaling triggered not by size changes in the granulocyte-macrophage population but by entry of foreign organisms to the body. Responses to foreign organisms could be quite complex. Even with the apparently simple CSF increases induced by the injection of endotoxin, there is now evidence that the CSF responses could depend on the prior production of other regulators, including IL-1 and/or tumor necrosis factor. In actual infections, it is even more likely that indirect mechanisms could be involved, with molecules released by damaged cells acting as mediators to elicit increased CSF synthesis by other cell types.

The CSF-producing system is therefore composed of widely dispersed cells of many types with an ability to respond very rapidly to emergencies such as acute infections by elevating CSF production. Exposure to microorganisms appears to be a major determinant of overall CSF production at any particular time. The elevation in levels of CSF and consequent activation of existing granulocyte-macrophage cells are rapid responses, and because of their speed, they almost certainly are important initial host responses to infections.

Intracellular Aspects of CSF Production

The synthesis of CSF by individual cells appears to follow the usual sequence of transcription of mRNA, translation, removal of the hydrophobic leader, and glycosylation followed by secretion through the membrane. There are, however, some unusual features of CSF synthesis: (1) the ability of cells to exhibit rapid changes of great magnitude in their rate of synthesis of CSF; (2) the possibility that some cells simultaneously produce two products, one for secretion and the other for membrane display; and (3) the ability of some cells to produce simultaneously more than one type of CSF. These features require some complexity in regulatory mechanisms, presumably both at the transcriptional and the translational level. Because quite different cell types are involved in CSF production, for example, fibroblasts versus lymphocytes, quite different mechanisms might be operating in different cells.

Studies on murine lymphocytes have shown that individual cells can produce at least two CSFs simultaneously, probably in addition to interferon, IL-5, and other biologically active macromolecules, following a single inductive membrane signal such as concanavalin A or binding of antibodies to the T-cell receptor. Similarly, fibroblasts can produce M-CSF, GM-CSF, and possibly some G-CSF after retroviral infection.

Within lymphocytes the increase in transcriptional activity is not exactly synchronous, and increases occur in GM-CSF transcription before that for Multi-CSF. Nevertheless, there is a strong presumption that initiating signals for transcription of these various macromolecules may be common, and a common potential initiation sequence is present adjacent to the relevant genes. The ability of fibroblasts to produce some but not all of these molecules following inductive signaling indicates either that a different signal is used in fibroblasts or that programing in the genome for CSF production is strongly influenced by cellular differentiation.

The possibility that certain cells might synthesize CSF for both secretion and membrane display has been raised by evidence indicating that stromal cells can secrete CSF but that hemopoiesis in long-term cultures seems to occur preferentially in contact with underlying stromal cells. The simplest suggestion for combining the two sets of observations is to postulate that the CSFs can be displayed on the membranes of some stromal cells. There is some evidence that this might be possible at least for M-CSF. Another interesting possibility arises from the demonstration that the glycohalix of stromal cells can bind CSFs and may function as the material in an affinity column, holding locally produced or humoral CSFs in a mode able to stimulate adjacent hemopoietic cells. A trivial explanation that has not yet been fully excluded is that the hemopoietic cell contact with certain cells in stromal layers is an artefact due to sedimentation of the hemopoietic cells plus a selectivity of binding to certain cells based on particular cell adhesion molecules not directly related to the control of hemopoiesis.

Neither lymphocytes nor fibroblasts express membrane receptors for the CSFs. However, in the case of normal monocyte-macrophages and certain transformed hemopoietic cells it can be shown that cells can simultaneously synthesize both CSF and CSF receptors. The implications of this situation for the development of leukemia will be discussed in Chapter 10. It is not known how compartmentalized a cytoplasm is in terms of its ability to segregate multiple polypeptide products, but it seems possible that where a cell synthesizes both CSF and CSF receptors, opportunities will occur for binding of these two products in a manner able to initiate signaling cascades. This seems a potentially dangerous situation for a normal cell, and intracellular systems may exist to minimize this possibility.

The capacity of cells to exhibit rapid induction of CSF synthesis in response to appropriate signaling makes it difficult to establish which cell types have no capacity to synthesize CSF under any circumstances. This problem is accentuated by the equally rapid decline in such induced synthetic activity. Most studies have been performed on normal cells, and it could be argued that such information inevitably underestimates the capacity of various cells. Thus normal skin cells display no apparent capacity to produce CSF, yet after exposure to phorbol esters, they clearly do produce CSF. Similarly, normal fibroblasts appear to produce only M-CSF, yet retrovirally infected fibroblasts not only increase the levels of M-CSF production but also produce detectable levels of GM-CSF and G-CSF.

Extension of these observations makes it possible to speculate that perhaps *all* tissue cell types may be able to produce one or another type of CSF if appropriately stimulated. The possibility that some cells might produce only small levels of CSF that remain intracytoplasmic makes it exceedingly difficult to establish whether granulocyte-macrophage cells might not on occasion produce their own CSF. Thus if microenvironmental cells function by inducing intracytoplasmic CSF in the target granulocytes and macrophages in contact with them, this process could be extremely difficult to detect other than by in situ hybridization. Furthermore, if physical disruption of the contact between stromal and target cells was quickly followed by decline of CSF transcription, active transcription might be undetectable in studies on purified populations of this type.

Half-Life and Fate of the CSFs

There are no methods available at present for determining the fate of a molecule produced locally in a tissue and eventually degraded or utilized at that site. The only current information on the fate of the CSFs is derived from studies on circulating CSF, and it should be kept in mind that locally produced molecules could be handled in a quite different manner. This comment may apply particularly to membrane-displayed CSF molecules.

When CSF is injected intravenously in the mouse, there is a rapid initial fall in CSF levels due in part to tissue equilibration, followed by a slower, second-phase decline. For the various CSFs the half-life of the first phase is 1 to 3 minutes, and that of the second phase 0.5 to 2 hours (Figure 29). These are fairly typical half-lives for glycoproteins of this type. In higher species the half-lives appear to be somewhat longer than those in the mouse, but the CSFs remain relatively short-lived molecules. The short serum half-lives, coupled with the ability of tissues to rapidly increase and decrease their rates of CSF synthesis, make the CSF system highly responsive and labile; major rises and falls in CSF levels can occur within hours.

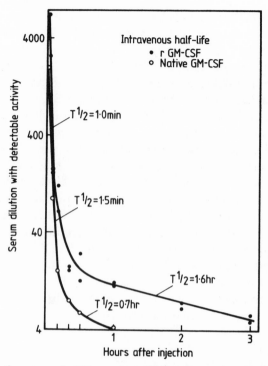

Figure 29. Similar serum half-lives of purified native and recombinant murine GM-CSF after intravenous injection into adult mice. With both there is an initial rapid fall followed by a second phase in which levels fall more slowly.

Studies using ^{125}I-labeled CSF indicate that although some injected CSF is cleared by the kidney, the large majority of the labeled material in the urine is degraded low-molecular-weight material. Autoradiography indicates rapid labeling of many tissues following the injection of ^{125}I CSF. From the functional viewpoint, the most important fact established is that such material does bind to hemopoietic cells in the marrow and spleen; therefore circulating CSF can be shown to be genuinely hormonal in nature since the molecules do have access to, and bind to, appropriate target cells. This was of interest because it had been suggested that since the marrow cell populations are tightly packed, circulating macromolecules might not obtain access to cells in such crowded tissues.

In quantitative terms, the majority of injected labeled CSF initially becomes localized in the liver, and shortly afterward the kidney contains the highest absolute levels of injected material. It cannot be certified that the labeling in such organs represents undegraded [125]I

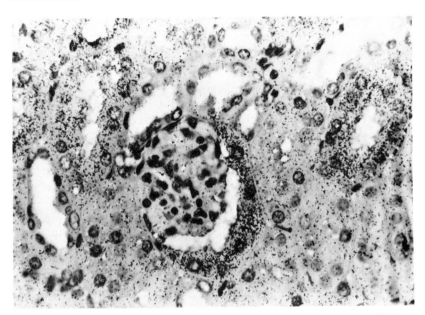

Figure 30. Autoradiograph of kidney tissue 1 hour after the intravenous injection of ^{125}I-labeled G-CSF. Note the intense labeling of cells of the Bowman's capsule and proximal renal tubules.

CSF, and in this context the thyroid of recipient mice becomes heavily labeled presumably by iodide released from degraded ^{125}I CSF. If it is assumed that the grains seen in autoradiographs do represent CSF, then in the liver the CSF is concentrated in endothelial and Kupffer cells. In the kidney a characteristic distribution is seen, with little labeling of the glomeruli but heavy labeling of Bowman's capsule cells and cells of the proximal renal tubules (Figure 30). This pattern of localization and the appearance shortly afterward in the urine of large amounts of low-molecular-weight radiolabeled material lead to the provisional conclusion that most injected CSF is degraded in the liver and kidney.

Why this should be so and why the process should be so rapid are unclear. It is usually postulated that glycoproteins are cleared by carbohydrate recognition, but recombinant bacterially synthesized (carbohydrate-free) CSFs are handled in a similar manner to the glycosylated native molecules. Attempts to detect conventional CSF receptors on liver or kidney cells have been unsuccessful, and studies using synthetic CSF peptides may be needed to determine which epitopes are recognized by the clearance mechanism.

Where cells bind CSF using specific membrane receptors (such as the granulocyte-macrophage population), the molecules are internalized with the receptor and little free CSF is subsequently released from the cell. The internalized CSF can be assumed to be degraded mainly by proteolytic systems. Breakdown of internalized CSF is not particularly rapid for most CSFs, and this route of breakdown would seem to be a quantitatively minor one. However, M-CSF is characterized by very rapid degradation, at least following internalization by certain types of macrophage. This has led to the suggestion that the entire fate of M-CSF in the body could be accounted for by degradation by tissue macrophages after M-CSF binding to specific membrane receptors. No autoradiographic studies appear to have been performed to determine the degree to which M-CSF is degraded in the liver and kidney, however, and it would be somewhat surprising for the metabolic fate of this CSF to differ so radically from that of the others.

More prolonged serum half-lives can be achieved by injecting CSF intraperitoneally or subcutaneously, but this presumably is the consequence of continuing entry of CSF into the circulation from the injection site. Little is known about whether carrier proteins for CSFs might exist in the serum.

Summary

The situation regarding CSF production in the body is quite complex. These molecules are clearly not the exclusive products of hemopoietic tissues and certainly not the exclusive products of granulocyte-macrophage populations themselves, even though at least one mature member of this population, the macrophage, does have an undoubted capacity to produce CSFs.

At a minimum, CSFs are produced throughout the tissues of the body; the major remaining uncertainty is whether they are products of all cells or merely of a variety of cells with a widespread distribution in all tissues.

The responsiveness of CSF synthesis to inductive signaling indicates that the ability of particular cells to produce CSF can only be determined by tests using a wide variety of experimental situations, and it can be presumed that our present knowledge underestimates this capacity even for cells that are readily accessible for testing.

The combination of the relatively short half-lives of the CSFs together with the extreme lability of CSF synthesis rates means that this regulatory system is a highly dynamic one capable of rapid and quantitatively large fluctuations in levels—a system designed admirably for rapid responses to a wide variety of emergency situations involving a need for the specialized functions of granulocyte-macrophage populations.

6

Modulators of CSF Action

In principle, the effects of any stimulus operating on a cell population could be modulated by either enhancers or inhibitors. Because the CSFs act mainly on progenitor cells and their progeny, any factor increasing the generation or responsiveness of progenitor cells is likely to enhance the final effects of CSF action. Conversely, the existence and mode of action of inhibitors of the CSFs are questions of particular importance because it is usually thought that a superior control system should include balancing inhibitors able to modulate the effects of proliferative stimuli.

Inhibitors of CSF Action

A variety of cell types could conceivably be sources of inhibitors able to reduce or suppress the effects of CSF stimulation. Such inhibitors could be products of the mature granulocytes and macrophages, of other hemopoietic cells such as stromal cells, of scattered specialized cells in various tissues, or of all cell types in the body.

A number of possible inhibitors could be envisaged: (1) factors suppressing CSF production; (2) factors making granulocyte-macrophage populations refractory to stimulation by CSF; (3) factors leading to accelerated breakdown or clearance of CSF; or (4) factors leading to accelerated death of mature granulocyte and macrophage populations or to a reduction in their functional activity. It would be reasonable to expect candidate inhibitors to be as lineage-restricted as the CSFs, and that their levels should be as labile as those of the CSFs.

Work with inhibitors based solely on the use of in vitro culture systems is notoriously prone to the risks of nonspecificity or detection of quite trivial phenomena. Changes in temperature, pH, or levels of metabolites that are nonlimiting in vivo may all produce dramatic inhibitory effects on cells proliferating in vitro yet be of no likely significance in vivo. Unfortunately, much of the present evidence on inhibitors has come from in vitro studies, and for many there is lack of clear evidence of specificity of action. None of the inhibitors thus far described resemble the CSFs in general biochemical nature. Although there is no particular reason why genuine inhibitors need resemble their agonists physically, the failure of the candidate inhibitors to remotely resemble the CSFs, often coupled with lack of convincing evidence of specificity, gives them a certain untidiness that falls far short of an elegant agonist-antagonist pharmacological system. There is also lack of evidence that the various candidate inhibitors interact in a concerted manner, as might be expected of a sophisticated control system.

It is not possible to group these inhibitors according to their biological actions; they will be discussed simply in terms of whether or not they originate from hemopoietic cells.

Intrinsic Inhibitors

The most elegant possibility is that products of mature granulocytes and macrophages themselves suppress granulocyte-macrophage proliferation, thereby directly ensuring some stability in total granulocyte-macrophage population size. There are four candidate inhibitors in this category, described in the following sections.

Prostaglandin E (PGE). This is one of the more interesting candidate inhibitors, although it has a diversity of actions in vivo. PGE is a product of monocyte-macrophages, and PGE production by such cells is enhanced by CSF stimulation. In vitro studies indicate that low concentrations (10^{-10} to 10^{-9} M) of PGE have a selective suppressing effect on macrophage colony formation, leaving granulocyte proliferation virtually unaltered. It is of further interest that PGE fails to inhibit the proliferation of macrophage precursors in chronic myeloid leukemic (CML) populations; thus a potential mechanism is offered for the unrestrained expansion exhibited by CML populations in vivo. There is some evidence indicating that only Ia-positive macrophage progenitors are suceptible to inhibition by PGE, which appears to block their entry into cell cycle. PGE appears not to be inhibitory for unrelated hemopoietic populations and thus to exhibit a certain selectivity for granulocyte-macrophage precursors.

Lactoferrin. This is another interesting candidate, since the molecule is a product of mature polymorphs. Lactoferrin has been reported to suppress CSF production by at least some cells but not to have a direct inhibitory effect on granulocyte-macrophage precursors themselves.

Granulocytic chalone. A hemoregulatory peptide (PGlu-Glu-Asp-Cys-Lys) that inhibits granulocyte-macrophage formation in vitro has been synthesized and an apparently similar peptide reported to be extractable from granulocyte-enriched populations. Although some evidence has been obtained for selectivity of action for granulocyte-macrophage populations, it is unclear whether this molecule exists in significant concentrations in the serum or tissues and whether levels fluctuate during perturbations in granulocyte-macrophage proliferation.

Macromolecular inhibitors. Extracts of bone marrow from various species have been found to inhibit entry of CFU-S into S-phase and have been postulated as inhibitors of hemopoiesis. Estimates of molecular weight indicate the possibility of two distinct inhibitors; one is of molecular weight less than 2,000 and may be the hemoregulatory peptide, while the second is estimated to be of molecular weight 30,000–50,000. It is difficult to conceive how factors acting only on stem cells might represent selective inhibitors of granulocyte-macrophage proliferation, since no mechanism presents itself for securing selectivity of action on granulocyte-macrophage populations.

In addition to these four inhibitors, hemopoietic cells themselves can exhibit a strain-based refractoriness to stimulation. Granulocyte-macrophage progenitors from certain mouse strains, for example, C57BL, appear more highly responsive to stimulation in vitro by CSF than do others, for example BALB/c. The basis for this differing responsiveness—whether receptor number differences, preexposure to modulating factors in vivo, or other mechanisms—is not yet known.

Extrinsic Inhibitors

Serum lipoproteins. Addition of serum from many mouse strains to cultures of mouse bone marrow cells inhibits granulocyte-macrophage colony formation. Fractionation of such sera indicated the inhibitory material to be lipoprotein in nature, with a molecular weight of about 250,000. Starvation of mice or preinjection with lipolytic heparin reduces the inhibitory activity of the serum. Comparable serum inhibitors have been detected in human sera, but the ability to detect these is strongly dependent on the batch of fetal calf serum used in the culture medium. Inhibitor levels were found to be abnormally low in about half of all samples tested from patients with acute myeloid leukemia and were low in sera from irradiated mice immediately prior to the onset of hemopoietic regeneration.

Although the data present some evidence of fluctuating inhibitor levels in situations of abnormal granulocyte-macrophage proliferation, there are aspects of the data that cast doubt on the significance of these serum inhibitors. There is no evidence of lineage-specificity; inhibition has also been observed of colony formation by unrelated lymphoid cells and cells of a variety of neoplastic cell lines. If inhibitors are concentrated so that the final concentration in the cultures equals that in normal serum, no granulocyte-macrophage proliferation is possible, regardless of the CSF concentration used. Preincubation of marrow cells with inhibitors results in selective macrophage colony formation when the cells are subsequently cultured in agar medium. Although there is some correlation between high inhibitor levels in certain mouse strains and a tendency for preferential macrophage colony formation by marrow cells from these strains, it is difficult to conceive how granulocyte and macrophage formation occurs in these mice if the in vitro data apply in vivo. It is necessary to postulate that granulocyte-macrophage populations in vivo are shielded from these inhibitory lipoproteins; otherwise no proliferation could occur. If this is indeed the explanation, it raises doubts about whether the inhibitors play any real role in controlling granulocyte-macrophage populations in vivo.

Enhancers of CSF Action

Three agents have been described with enhancing effects on CSF action.

IL-1. A series of studies showed that media conditioned by certain tissues or cell lines were able to increase the number of granulocyte-macrophage progenitor cells particularly in marrow populations from mice pretreated with the cytotoxic agent 5-FU and depleted of cycling precursors, including most progenitor cells. The active factor was termed hemopoietin I, or enhancing factor, and was purified to homogeneity from media conditioned by the human bladder cancer cell line 5637. Use of specific antisera has suggested that this molecule is in fact interleukin-I (IL-1), a molecule characterized initially as inducing expression of IL-2 receptors on T-lymphocytes and allowing responsiveness of these cells to stimulation by IL-2.

Hemopoietin I (IL-1) also induces enhanced expression of M-CSF receptors on primitive hemopoietic stem cells and their immediate progeny, accentuating their proliferation when stimulated by M-CSF. Since this potentiating action of hemopoietin I on cellular proliferation has also been observed when it is used in combination with GM-CSF, G-CSF, and Multi-CSF, it seems possible that IL-1 may be able to induce membrane expression of a quite broad range of specific receptor molecules on appropriate precursor cells. The net effect of this action is to permit the CSFs to stimulate the proliferation of larger numbers of potential precursor cells, including quite primitive cells with very high proliferative potential. As mentioned earlier, injected IL-1 is also able to elicit serum increases in CSF levels.

Corticosteroids. Hydrocortisone and cortisone have complex effects. Injection of mice with cortisone causes a fall in circulating CSF levels, while addition of hydrocortisone to cultures selectively enhances granulocyte colony formation and appears to be essential for the formation of granulocyte colonies in serum-free cultures. Cortisone has also been described as altering the responsiveness of the granulocyte-macrophage progenitors to stimulation by CSF in vitro.

fMet-Leu-Phe. This peptide is a chemotactic agent for polymorphs and is believed to be released from both microorganisms and damaged tissues. Studies on the binding of radiolabeled G-CSF to mature granulocytes showed that preexposure of the cells to fMet-Leu-Phe down-modulated binding of G-CSF. Since fMet-Leu-Phe can also stimulate some functional activities of mature granulocytes, its ability to down-modulate G-CSF receptors may indicate an ability to mimic or potentiate the activating effects of G-CSF.

Summary

It is perhaps natural that information on modulators of CSF action has lagged behind that on the CSFs themselves. In view of the diverse cellular origins of the CSFs, researchers investigating inhibitors of CSF action may have concentrated their attention unduly on granulocyte and macrophage populations. The biology of the CSFs suggests that significant inhibitors could be products of almost any tissue in the body. There is also a profound lack of information on fluctuations in the levels of candidate inhibitors in appropriate situations that would allow a prima facie case to be made for their possible importance in vivo.

As was the case with the CSFs, real progress in this field will depend on purification of adequate amounts of inhibitors and on the development of recombinant inhibitors to allow testing of their action in the intact body.

7

Actions of the CSFs In Vivo

During the twenty-year history of work on the CSFs as mandatory proliferative stimuli for granulocyte-macrophage proliferation in vitro, the proposition that the CSFs were genuine regulators of these populations in vivo had to be based on indirect evidence and argument by analogy.

The indirect evidence was strong, and it remains today an important part of the data permitting the conclusion that CSFs indeed are regulators in vivo. As discussed earlier, the indirect evidence is essentially the following: first, that the CSFs are detectable in serum and tissues in concentrations known to be active on granulocyte-macrophage cells in vitro, and second, that levels of CSF alter during infections and in perturbations of granulocyte-macrophage formation, as might be expected if they were responsible for regulating granulocyte-macrophage proliferation. Strong supporting evidence was also obtained from an analysis of animals and patients with tumors who were also exhibiting a granulocytosis. Investigation showed that such tumors contained and produced high levels of CSF, that serum CSF levels were elevated, and that the excess granulocyte levels returned to normal following resection of the tumor. The problem with the tumor data was that the effects may have been due to some other unknown product of tumor cells or may have been a host response to the presence of tumor tissue, mediated by some molecule other than CSF.

It seemed pointless to investigate the in vivo effects of injecting crude CSF-containing material because the effects could not be attributed with certainty to CSF. Furthermore, because of the in vitro dose-responses, the known short half-lives of the CSFs in vivo, and the very small amounts of purified CSF able to be extracted from even the richest tissue sources, there was no real prospect of being able to inject sufficient purified CSF into an animal to observe what responses were induced.

This somewhat gloomy prospect has been transformed by the advent of molecular biology and the demonstration that biologically active recombinant material can be produced in large amounts using mammalian, yeast, or bacterial expression systems. Careful comparative studies in vitro of native versus recombinant CSFs, particularly of nonglycosylated bacterially synthesized CSFs, have revealed no differences between recombinant and native CSFs in specific activity, range of target cell action, receptor binding affinities, or organ distribution in vivo. There may be differences in serum half-lives between glycosylated and nonglycosylated forms, but present data do not show these differences to be major in degree. Thus the production of recombinant CSFs has now allowed extensive studies on the effects of CSF in both normal and abnormal animals that have culminated in the present clinical trials of these molecules.

Based on in vitro data, there were certain expectations of what might be observable in vivo following the injection of different CSFs. To a large degree, the data from in vivo responses have been in remarkable agreement with expectations, but there have been some interesting differences. As shown in Figure 18, it is a familiar finding in mouse cultures that GM-CSF and Multi-CSF stimulate the formation of large numbers of large colonies, two-thirds of which are wholly or partly composed of granulocytic cells. In contrast, G-CSF appears to be a very weak proliferative stimulus, causing the formation of small numbers of colonies all of which are remarkably small in size. On this basis, G-CSF was anticipated to be likely to produce only moderate effects on granulocyte levels in vivo compared with those inducible by GM-CSF or Multi-CSF. However, the opposite has been observed. Furthermore, even though all in vitro studies indicated that G-CSF has no action on early erythroid progenitors and virtually no action on multipotential or stem cells, the injection of G-CSF in vivo produces remarkable changes in erythroid populations in the mouse. These discrepancies emphasize the complexity of the control systems operating on hemopoiesis in vivo and the opportunity for significant indirect effects to occur in vivo following the injection of a single active agent that perturbs an existing equilibrium. Although the mouse is the most convenient animal for a detailed analysis of in vivo effects, the need to obtain preclinical data and the species restrictions in cross-reactivity of the CSFs have necessitated extensive primate studies as well as studies in a wide range of species.

The types of responses observed are best illustrated by considering the effects in normal adult mice of GM-CSF, Multi-CSF, and G-CSF. Injection intraperitoneally of doses of 6 to 200 ng of purified, bacterially synthesized, recombinant, mouse-active CSF three times daily for 6 days produces clear dose-related responses with all three CSFs. The responses are comparable in C57BL, BALB/c, and the endotoxin-hyporesponsive strain C3H/HeJ mice. Although mice of all strains exhibit similar qualitative responses, the occurrence of strain-related differences in the magnitude of certain of the responses predicts that individual humans will also exhibit some differences in responses.

Responses in Hemopoietic Tissues

The Peripheral Blood

G-CSF is the most effective CSF in inducing increased polymorph levels in the peripheral blood (Figure 31), with levels rising from the normal level of 500 to 1,000 per microliter to more than 20,000 per microliter. If higher doses of G-CSF are used or the injection schedule is extended, levels up to 100,000 per microliter can be achieved. Only with high G-CSF concentrations are minor elevations in monocyte levels elicited, and no changes occur in eosinophil or lymphocyte levels. GM-CSF and Multi-CSF are ineffective in inducing substantial neutrophil increases in the mouse; the highest doses induce only a two- to three-fold elevation. Both GM-CSF and Multi-CSF induce a small elevation of monocyte and eosinophil levels. The minor changes induced by GM-CSF in mice are curious because in monkeys and man GM-CSF induces major elevations in blood neutrophil and eosinophil levels. Combination of G-CSF with GM-CSF in the mouse leads to an additive effect on peripheral blood cell levels.

Increases induced by G-CSF can be sustained for several weeks without evidence of depletion of precursors or the development of a refractory state.

The peripheral-blood neutrophil increases are progressive with time, and although they become evident by 24 hours, the kinetics suggest they are the consequence of increased cell production rather than of cell release or redistribution from existing tissue pools. However, G-CSF does appear to have some direct or indirect neutrophil-

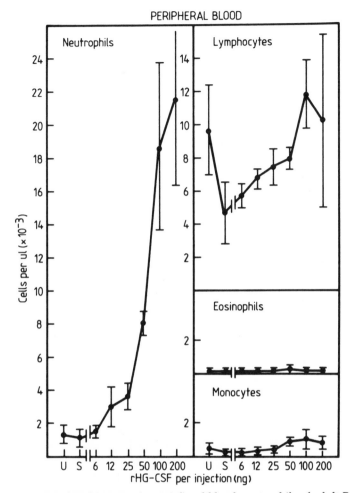

Figure 31. Dose-related increase in peripheral-blood neutrophils of adult BALB/c mice injected three times daily for 6 days with doses of from 6 to 200 ng rG-CSF. Mice were analyzed on day 7.

releasing action since moderate increases are demonstrable within hours of injection, and these cells are unlikely to represent newly formed cells.

The Peritoneal Cavity

The intraperitoneal injection of all three CSFs induces a progressive rise with time in cellularity in the peritoneal cavity with little evidence

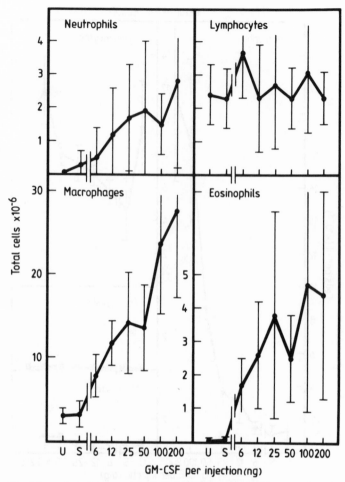

Figure 32. Dose-related increases in peritoneal macrophages, eosinophils, and neutrophils of adult BALB/c mice injected intraperitoneally three times daily for 6 days with doses of from 6 to 200 ng rGM-CSF. Mice were analyzed on day 7.

of rapid migration into the cavity of preexisting cells, as monitored at 3 or 6 hours after a single injection. The quantitatively largest cellular response involves peritoneal macrophages, and the most effective agent in eliciting such rises is GM-CSF (Figure 32). After 6 days of stimulation by GM-CSF, levels of macrophages have been observed as high as 100×10^6, as compared with the normal number of 1–2×10^6. Levels of macrophages achieved by Multi-CSF seem to plateau at less than 20×10^6 and with G-CSF rarely exceed 10×10^6 per mouse.

The peritoneal macrophages of a CSF-injected mouse are larger and more basophilic than normal macrophages and exhibit heightened mitotic activity, particularly in the first few days of the response to CSF injection. Calculations show that the increased local mitotic activity would be sufficient to account for about half the observed increase in the macrophages in mice injected with GM-CSF.

All three CSFs also induce increases in peritoneal neutrophils; again GM-CSF and Multi-CSF are more effective than G-CSF. These cells are exclusively postmitotic and must have migrated into the peritoneal cavity from the circulation. GM-CSF and Multi-CSF, but not G-CSF, also elicit increases in peritoneal eosinophils, again without evidence of local proliferation.

Although intraperitoneal injection of CSFs induces the highest rise in peritoneal cellularity and thus could be eliciting a purely local response, in fact some increase in peritoneal cellularity can be elicited by the subcutaneous injection of CSF, indicating that the response is in part a systemic one.

The macrophages in mice injected with GM-CSF frequently exhibit phagocytosis of eosinophils, and tests on peritoneal macrophages from mice injected with GM-CSF and Multi-CSF indicate that the CSFs induce substantial increases in the proportion of phagocytically active cells and in the number of antibody-coated erythroid cells phagocytosed per cell. Injection of GM-CSF combined with G-CSF produces an enhancement of increases in peritoneal cell numbers, particularly in the case of neutrophils.

The Spleen

Because the normal mouse marrow is tightly packed with cells, no expansion of total marrow cell numbers can occur. In the mouse, therefore, the spleen is the organ exhibiting responsiveness to increased hemopoiesis by increases in weight, cellularity, and the proportion of hemopoietic versus lymphoid cells. Injection of all three CSFs for 6 days increases spleen weight, the increases ranging from 50 percent with GM-CSF to 300 percent with G-CSF. A clear rise is observed in the spleen content of granulocytic cells only with G-CSF. With Multi-CSF and the higher doses of GM-CSF, a dose-related rise is observed in spleen megakaryocytes, in agreement with the known actions of these two molecules in vitro. Of the four CSFs, only Multi-

CSF has proliferative effects on mast cells in vitro, and in agreement with this finding, only Multi-CSF induces increases in spleen mast cells (Figure 33). In appropriate strains, this increase is extremely large (more than 100-fold) and involves mainly incompletely granulated cells. A characteristic location of these increased mast cells is the sinus region around the spleen lymphoid follicles, an observation of interest because this is the location of cells with exceptionally high numbers of receptors for Multi-CSF. Since the increased numbers of mast cells in this location often occur in clonal-like aggregates, these high-receptor-bearing cells may be the precursors of such clones.

Because Multi-CSF was known from in vitro studies to be able to stimulate the proliferation of stem cells and the formation of progenitor cells from stem cells, it was not surprising to observe a 10- to 30-fold elevation in the numbers of stem and progenitor cells in the spleen of mice injected with Multi-CSF. Again, since GM-CSF is weakly active on these populations in vitro, it was also not surprising to observe a 3- to 5-fold elevation of progenitor cell numbers in the spleen following injection of GM-CSF. However, G-CSF has no significant proliferative action in vitro on stem, multipotential, or erythroid progenitors, and it was quite unexpected to observe 10- to 50-fold elevations of the numbers of these cells in spleens of mice injected with G-CSF. Because G-CSF has no known in vitro action in stimulating erythropoiesis, it was also surprising that the enlarged spleen of mice injected with G-CSF contained up to 60 percent nucleated erythroid cells, a 30- to 40-fold rise in total spleen erythroid cells achieved within 7 days.

Bone Marrow

As already mentioned, the mouse marrow is normally tightly packed and cannot increase its total cell numbers. In mice injected with Multi-CSF or G-CSF, total marrow cell numbers remain constant but there is a progressive dose-related rise in the proportion of granulocytic cells, particularly in mice injected with G-CSF. This rise occurs at the expense of the lymphoid and erythroid populations, which fall to extremely low levels. In mice injected with GM-CSF, the situation differs in that an actual fall occurs in total cell numbers but with a rise in the percentage of granulocytic cells. Total progenitor cell numbers remain constant in the marrow of mice injected with G-CSF or Multi-CSF but are somewhat reduced in mice injected with GM-CSF.

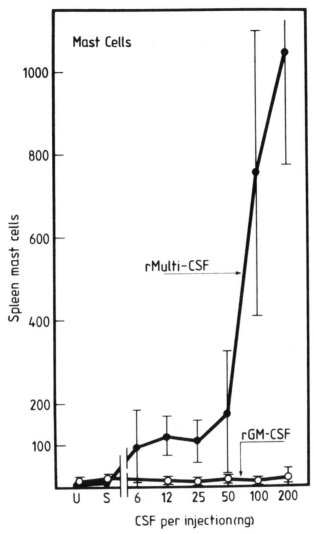

Figure 33. Dose-related increase in immature mast cells in the spleen of adult BALB/c mice injected three times daily for 6 days with doses of from 6 to 200 ng rMulti-CSF. Mice were examined on day 7.

Responses in Nonhemopoietic Tissues

Injection of CSF in mice results in a tendency for increased numbers of mature hemopoietic cells to accumulate in nonhemopoietic tissues. This is most readily documented by increases in the liver content of nonparenchymal cells, mainly monocytes, neutrophils, and eosinophils, in mice injected with Multi-CSF or GM-CSF. Increases in the lung content of granulocytes and monocytes are also observed in mice injected with GM-CSF, while 2- to 4-fold increases in mast cells are observed in the gut and skin of mice injected with Multi-CSF.

Responses in Other Species

Information on the response to injected CSF in other species is limited mainly to data on the peripheral white cell levels. However, in dogs, guinea pigs, primates, and humans injection of G-CSF or GM-CSF at doses approximately 5–20 μg per kilogram per day have been shown to increase neutrophil levels up to 50,000 per microliter, with a clear dose relationship between the amount of CSF injected and the level of neutrophils achieved.

Responses in Animals with Marrow Damage

Some of the most dramatic effects of injected CSF have been observed in animals whose marrow populations have been damaged by cytotoxic drugs or whole-body irradiation. Injection of G-CSF is able to diminish or prevent the cytopenia induced by cytotoxic drugs and accelerates the rate of regeneration. Similarly, injection of G-CSF or GM-CSF into irradiated primates given marrow transplants accelerates the regeneration of hemopoietic tissue and shortens the time elapsing before neutrophil levels in the peripheral blood attain clinically important levels (more than 1,000 per microliter). In dogs with cyclic neutropenia, the injection of G-CSF prevents the cyclical falls in neutrophil levels.

Summary

The studies in mice and other animals on the responses to injected CSF have clearly documented increases in total numbers of granulocytes and monocytes both in hemopoietic and nonhemopoietic tissues that vary in magnitude up to 100-fold. The inference is strong that these increases result from stimulation of granulocyte and macrophage formation (and of the formation of eosinophils, mast cells, and megakaryocytes for mice injected with Multi-CSF) and that injected CSF acts in vivo in the same manner as it does in vitro. This conclusion is supported by evidence of in vivo functional activation of macrophages identical in nature to that demonstrable following exposure of such cells to CSF in vitro.

Most of the observed responses are known from previous in vitro studies to be direct effects of the CSFs on the populations, and it seems unnecessary to postulate that the in vivo effects are achieved by other than direct effects of the injected CSF. However, a more complex interpretation is required to account for the unexpected effects of G-CSF on erythroid, stem, and multipotential progenitor cells. Since these effects do not correspond with known actions of G-CSF in vitro, some type of indirect effect must be initiated by the injection of this CSF, but the mechanism is unknown.

The data on the effects of injecting CSF into animals provide very strong support for the conclusion that CSFs are genuine regulators of granulocyte and macrophage formation in vivo. It is still possible, however, to question the completeness of the in vivo evidence. The data certainly show that the CSFs *can* regulate granulocyte-macrophage proliferation but do not actually prove that this is the normal manner in which this proliferation is regulated. Final proof of this proposition requires the use of anti-CSF antisera. If injection of such antisera in mice results in the depressed formation of granulocytes and macrophages, formal proof would be complete that the CSFs can and *do* regulate granulocyte and macrophage formation in vivo. Because of the antigenic differences among the four CSFs, it will be necessary to use a mixture of four types of antisera for this type of study.

8

Role of the CSFs in Resistance to Infections

Following the entry into the body of a highly pathogenic organism with a capacity for rapid replication, a life-threatening infection could develop within 24 to 48 hours unless the body is able to respond rapidly in a manner that either eliminates the organisms or localizes the infection. A century ago, clear evidence was obtained for the ability of the reticuloendothelial system to respond rapidly in such situations, but the importance accorded to this system declined with the preoccupation of immunologists with the elegant specificity of responses involving antibodies and T- and B-lymphocytes. Although the latter cells have an unquestioned involvement in resistance to acute infections, their limitation in an infection by an organism to which the body has not previously been exposed is the relative slowness with which immune responses develop. Since the body has an effective ability to resist acute infections, it seems likely that the initial defense is based on responses of the reticuloendothelial system.

For the purposes of this discussion, the reticuloendothelial system will be considered to include three major effector cell types, the polymorph, monocyte-macrophage, and eosinophil, acting in collaboration with endothelial cells and fibroblasts in an affected tissue. This system relies on an ability to mobilize, localize, and activate effector cells at the site of infection in an inflammatory response which, if effective, would prevent dissemination of organisms from the original site. In situations where elimination of organisms is not able to be achieved locally, the same cell populations would continue to resist the now disseminated organisms until the infection was overcome or until lymphocyte-based immune responses developed.

The key considerations for such a resistance system are the speed with which responses can be elicited and the efficiency with which existing effector cells can be localized and activated. Initially at least, an ability to amplify the number of such effector cells would not be important, although it would clearly be advantageous to produce additional effector cells as rapidly as possible if the infection persisted.

Consideration of the actions of the CSFs and the biology of CSF production indicates that this regulatory system is ideally suited to elicit ultrarapid responses in the relevant effector cell populations, as well as to control for extended periods the formation of additional effector cells. The expectation that CSFs are the primary mediators controlling resistance to infection is supported by survey evidence indicating that CSF levels are ultralow in germ-free animals, are higher in conventional animals, presumably with intermittent subclinical infections, and are extremely high during the acute phases of a wide variety of infections. As discussed earlier, the bacterial cell wall component endotoxin and a variety of bacterial products are potent inducers of CSF synthesis. Cells able to respond rapidly to endotoxin include endothelial cells and macrophages, the cells most likely to make initial contact with invading microorganisms. Studies on carrageenin-induced local inflammatory lesions have revealed a high CSF content in the fluid and active CSF production by cells surrounding the inflammatory sites. Tissues that are the site of infections have been found to produce large amounts of CSF.

Although the exact cells producing CSF in infectious foci have not been clearly identified, it is apparent that such tissues not only can promptly elevate local levels of CSF but can produce elevated systemic levels of CSF for sustained periods. Thus the CSF system fulfills the basic requirements of a primary response system—that responses be rapid, quantitatively large, and sustainable.

The ability of the CSFs to induce functional activation of mature neutrophils, monocytes, and eosinophils has been discussed earlier. These functional activation responses are also rapid in onset, being demonstrable within minutes of exposing cells to CSF, and are sustainable for prolonged periods, decaying only following withdrawal of CSF. The observed activations are exactly those likely to be relevant for effective responses to microorganisms, namely increased phagocytosis and intracellular killing, increased superoxide production, and increased production of macromolecules likely to be of relevance in eliciting local inflammatory responses, such as TNF, PGE, plasminogen activator, IL-1 production, and so forth. There is also evidence for the existence of signaling cascades that, in sites of local inflammation, could lead to progressive amplification of responses. For example, IL-1 can induce CSF synthesis, which itself elicits IL-1 production.

The CSFs therefore clearly possess the ability to activate effector cells to eliminate invading microorganisms, as well as the ability to elicit the production of other molecules likely to result in a progressive amplification of local cellular responses.

The CSFs have also been shown to have both chemotactic and immobilizing effects on polymorphs and monocytes, as well as an action leading to increased adherence of such cells. Although there is some evidence that the chemotactic effects may be direct actions, it is possible that they could also be mediated by indirect effects, particularly in vivo.

CSFs have also been shown to inhibit locomotion of effector cells, GM-CSF being identified as the factor previously described as neutrophil inhibitory factor (NIF). This action appears to compete with the chemotactic effects but could be based on responses elicited by differing CSF concentrations. It is conceivable that the two types of action could operate in concert, with lower CSF concentrations being chemotactic and attracting effector cells to an inflammatory site where the highest CSF concentration ensures retention of the cells by inhibiting further cell migration. This would be a highly efficient system for quickly building up high local concentrations of effector cells from populations previously dispersed throughout the body. It is likely that other macromolecules being released within inflammatory sites would also influence this concentration and localization of effector cells.

Thus the CSFs possess the second set of functional actions required to regulate rapid host responses, the ability to elicit accumulations of effector cells at the inflammatory site and to activate them functionally.

In situations where the nature of an infection is such that speedy elimination of organisms using existing effector cells does not occur and increased production of effector cells becomes of progressive importance, the CSFs clearly have the ability to regulate the increased production of granulocytes, macrophages, and eosinophils. Since increased serum CSF levels are a characteristic of acute infections, the tissues of the body have the capacity to provoke and sustain major elevations in tissue and circulating CSF levels. The ability of injected CSF to elevate neutrophil levels to extremely high levels attests to the capacity of these agents to elevate effector cell levels to those seen in most infections, and such elevations are able to be sustained for weeks.

Although it would be naive to attempt to attribute all facets of a complex antimicrobial response to a single set of regulatory molecules, the CSFs nevertheless seem to possess a surprisingly complete set of relevant functional activities, and this, coupled with an efficient system for rapidly modulating local or systemic levels of CSF, seems to indicate a central role of the CSFs in acute resistance to infections.

Information is meager on the exact type of CSF involved in such local or systemic responses. More precise information from model infections may require the use of in situ hybridization probes together with more careful analysis of the CSF types in inflammatory fluid.

The consideration of the requirements for effective rapid responses to invading microorganisms and the ability of the CSFs to mediate the necessary cellular events could be summarized by examining the possible events in two differing clinical situations.

Transient infections. Invasion of a capillary by microorganisms might elicit immediate CSF release by adjacent capillary endothelial and fibroblast cells, with the rapid accumulation of a high local concentration of CSF (Figure 34). Circulating neutrophils and monocytes could be attracted to this region, localized by the action of the CSFs, and functionally activated to eliminate the organisms. This whole process could be complete within minutes or at most hours, with little clinical evidence of an infection having occurred.

Sustained infections. Bacterial pneumonia in the preantibiotic days might be a possible model of this type of situation. Resolution of the infection was known to be dependent on the development of adequately elevated neutrophil levels and the sequential invasion and accumulation in the lung of neutrophils and then monocyte-macrophages, which eliminated the organisms and removed the attendant products of tissue damage. In this kind of situation, local production of CSFs by the lung would be expected to be high, leading to attraction of polymorphs and monocytes to the diseased lung and their functional activation (Figure 35). The extensiveness of the infection would result in major increases in serum CSF levels due to CSF production not only in the lung but throughout the body. These high CSF levels would stimulate increased production of granulocytes and

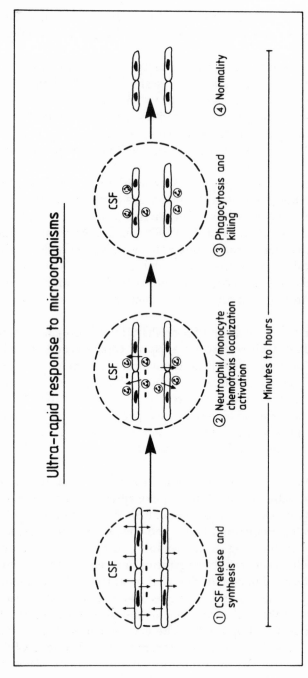

Figure 34. Possible events terminating an infection in its earliest phase. Bacterial products trigger local CSF release; the high CSF levels attract and then activate effector cells, eliminating the infecting microorganisms.

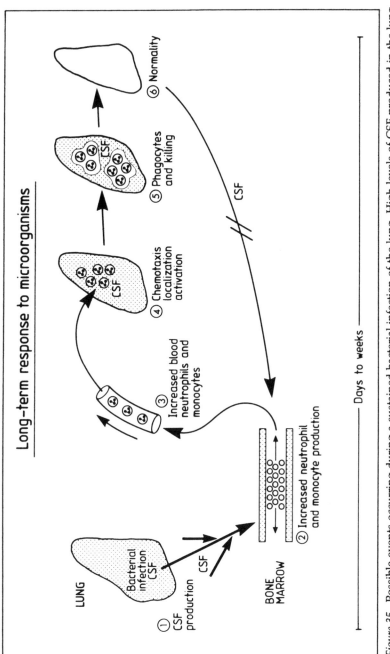

Figure 35. Possible events occurring during a sustained bacterial infection of the lung. High levels of CSF produced in the lung and other tissues stimulate the formation of additional neutrophils and monocytes. The high lung CSF levels attract, localize, and activate these cells in the lung, eliminating the infection and removing damaged cells. The system returns to normal with elimination of the microorganisms enhancing CSF production.

monocytes, with elevated circulating levels of these cells allowing amplification of the local responses in the lung. Resolution of the infection would remove the signals for increased CSF production, and, given the short half-lives of the CSFs, the granulocyte-macrophage system would quickly return to basal levels of both cell production and mature cell activation. In view of the exceptional ability of G-CSF to stimulate neutrophil responses, at least in mice, it is of interest that G-CSF elevation is so prominent in the serum in acute responses to endotoxin injection and infections.

The situation with viral or protozoal infections is less clear-cut. Elevated CSF levels have been observed following viral infections, but in most cases secondary bacterial infections may also have been present; thus it is unclear whether resolution of a simple viral infection necessarily involves CSF-mediated responses. The fact that T-lymphocytes have been shown to be necessary for such responses does not eliminate the involvement of granulocyte-macrophage responses, because changes in these latter populations do occur in the acute phases of viral infections and activated T-lymphocytes produce GM-CSF and Multi-CSF, at least in vitro.

For protozoal infections there is clear evidence that T-lymphocytes are necessary for cellular responses and that GM-CSF can activate killing of schistosomula by eosinophils, so again the CSFs, whether or not of T-lymphocyte origin, could play an important role in some aspects of resistance to infections of this type.

There are also chronic infections such as leishmaniasis or lepromatous leprosy in which monocytes play an obvious, if often incomplete, role. In principle, such monocytic responses should in part at least be CSF-dependent. This is of obvious potential relevance for the problem of inadequate host responses in chronic infections and is in need of further exploration.

If there is any substance in these proposals that the CSFs are of central importance in mediating resistance to infections, particularly in the acute stages, then it should be demonstrable that the injection of CSF significantly enhances resistance to test infections using either bacteria or fungi. Studies have now been performed in mice on this question using both G-CSF and GM-CSF. Test animals were either normal or pretreated with cytotoxic drugs to damage hemopoietic tissues prior to challenge with lethal doses of either bacteria or yeast organisms. In both types of test animals the injection of CSFs substantially enhanced resistance, permitting survival of infected mice with challenge doses up to 1,000-fold higher than those killing control animals.

Summary

These impressive responses, particularly in compromised animals, using the types of organisms common in clinical situations (for example, pseudomonas or candida) suggest that the use of CSFs in patients with similar life-threatening infections may result in a substantial enhancement of resistance and survival. If these expectations can be confirmed by present clinical trials, then the CSFs will represent nontoxic agents of great potential value for use in association with conventional antibiotic therapy, particularly for infections where adequate antimicrobial agents do not exist, such as fungal infections.

Because at least G-CSF and GM-CSF elicit characteristically different patterns of cellular response, it would be logical to envisage the combined use of such CSFs, thereby copying the responses in natural infections where elevations of more than one type of CSF occur. Thus for a patient with a peritoneal infection following bowel surgery, local infusion of GM-CSF into the peritoneal cavity coupled with the systemic administration of G-CSF would capitalize on the features of both types of response and should allow optimal stimulation of host responses.

Consideration must be given to whether the use of such natural regulators should be restricted only to uncommon life-threatening infections or whether they could be usefully employed for more common if somewhat trivial infections such as recurrent sinusitis, perhaps by local administration. Much hinges on whether the recombinant CSFs prove to be antigenic in man, whether such antibodies limit continuing responses, and, above all, whether the antibodies cross-inhibit native CSFs. If antibody production should emerge as a significant problem, clearly it would be irresponsible to use such agents for other than rare life-threatening infections.

A common clinical problem in which the use of CSFs may possibly prove to be valuable occurs in patients with depressed hemopoiesis as a result of treatment of cancers with cytotoxic drugs and in patients with ablated bone marrow receiving marrow transplants. In both situations, the occurrence of infections during the period of resulting neutropenia can be either disabling or fatal. In experimental animals, the injection of CSF can either prevent the development of neutropenia or shorten the subsequent period of neutropenia by a significant amount. In these situations where infections can be anticipated, the use of CSFs could be regarded as being prophylactic; and even if they do not actually prevent infections, the CSFs have the possible ability to transform a clinically apparent infection to a subclinical infection of brief duration and low morbidity.

Whether there is value in extending this concept of prophylaxis to procedures notoriously prone to infective complications, such as bowel surgery, will depend on information about the effectiveness of CSF therapy and the risks involved in possibly generating anti-CSF antibodies.

9

Toxic Effects of the CSFs

Whether the CSFs prove to have any acute toxic effects after infusion into humans will become apparent from clinical trials in progress. Certain biological mediators such as IL-1, tumor necrosis factor, and γ-interferon, some of whose levels rise in acute infections, have been observed to have a miscellany of toxic effects, which suggests that they may be responsible in part for the malaise associated with acute infections. Although the CSFs, as normally occurring hormones, are less likely to induce comparable effects, CSF levels are substantially elevated in infections and it is conceivable that at high concentrations the CSFs might also induce some minor symptoms.

A more substantial potential problem arises in situations in which elevated CSF levels are maintained for an extended period. Because of the ability of the CSFs to stimulate end cell functional activity, it is possible that toxic levels of products of such cells could induce either local or systemic damage in various tissues. This applies particularly to products of monocytes and macrophages, since these cells can produce a number of potentially damaging molecules. Preliminary information that long-term exposure to high CSF levels may have damaging effects on other tissues has come from an analysis of transgenic mice bearing two additional copies of the GM-CSF gene linked to the Moloney virus LTR promoter. Such mice constitutively express grossly elevated serum levels of GM-CSF (2,000 to 3,000 units per milliliter versus less than 50 units per milliliter in litter-mate control mice).

A curious feature of these transgenic mice relates to the appearance of GM-CSF in the urine. Two lines of transgenic mice were established; in one of these lines (female-derived) insertion is on the X chromosome, whereas the insertion site in the other line (male-derived) is on an unidentified autosomal chromosome. High GM-CSF levels equal to or exceeding those in the serum were observed in the urine of male mice of the male-derived line. However, despite the fact that serum GM-CSF levels were similar in the other transgenic mice, little or no GM-CSF was observed in the urine either of female mice of the male-derived line or of males or females of the female-derived line.

These mice do not exhibit prenatal or neonatal morbidity and are apparently healthy until 2 months of age. After this time, however, mice begin to die, with progressive weight loss, muscle wasting, and tremors. All mice of the female-derived line are dead by 5 months of age, as are 50 percent of mice of the male-derived line. From birth, the transgenic mice are readily identifiable because of ocular opacity. The basis for this opacity is the presence within both chambers of the eye of activated macrophages which, within weeks, induce blindness by retinal destruction with some cataractogenous changes in the lens.

Although appearing healthy as young adult mice, transgenic GM-CSF mice in fact exhibit dramatic accumulations of activated macrophages in both the peritoneal and pleural cavities, with levels in the peritoneal cavity reaching as high as 500×10^6 versus a normal number of $1-2 \times 10^6$. Elevated numbers of eosinophils and neutrophils are also present in these locations. This cellular response is reminiscent of the changes induced in normal mice by the intraperitoneal injection of GM-CSF. Oddly, but again in line with the response of mice to injected GM-CSF, white cell levels in the peripheral blood are not elevated, although in occasional mice a few activated macrophages are seen in the blood.

The organs of the abdominal and pleural cavities are coated with masses of activated macrophages, which do not, however, penetrate the organ capsules. With time, organizing fibrous tissue develops on the surface of these organs in the interface between the organ capsule and the surrounding macrophages, and the fibrous tissue comes to contain substantial numbers of eosinophils, neutrophils, and lymphocytes. In some mice this organizing fibrous tissue forms nodules on the diaphragm and other organs, with some penetration of organ capsules.

These mice develop a progressive diffuse and focal cellular infiltration in all striated muscle tissue (Figure 36) and less commonly in nonstriated muscle such as the heart. Initially the infiltrating cells are mainly activated macrophages, but with time, eosinophils, neutrophils, lymphocytes, and fibroblasts also appear. This cellular infiltra-

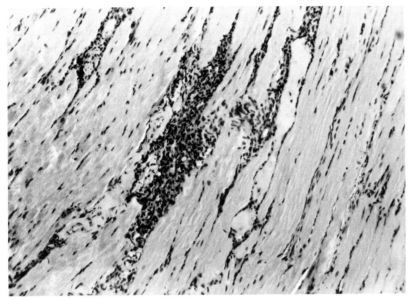

Figure 36. Foci of activated macrophages and other cells in muscle tissue from a transgenic GM-CSF mouse dying with wasting and muscle tremors.

tion is associated with degeneration of adjacent muscle cells and appears to be the likely cause of the progressive muscular damage and weakness preceding death.

The origin of the excess macrophages has yet to be determined and is puzzling since normal numbers of granulocyte-macrophage progenitors are present in the marrow and spleen of transgenic mice. Furthermore, these progenitor cells generate colonies of normal size and composition in vitro and exhibit a normal absolute dependency on extrinsic CSF for proliferation in vitro, and indeed a normal quantitative responsiveness to recombinant GM-CSF during colony formation. There is no suggestion from their behavior in culture that cells are either autonomous or neoplastic, a conclusion confirmed by the lack of mitotic activity in vivo of the enlarged activated macrophages.

That the transgenic macrophages are functionally activated is attested by their increased phagocytic activity for antibody-coated sheep erythrocytes. Indeed, some mice show extensive erythrocytic phagocytosis in vivo with accompanying splenomegaly, the spleen containing large numbers of nucleated erythroid cells.

Information on the tissues expressing the transgene is incomplete, but in adult mice, tissues known to express mRNA for the transgene are peritoneal macrophages, eye tissue, and muscle tissue. An interesting observation regarding the transgenic macrophages is that despite chronic exposure to high GM-CSF levels, they continue to express membrane receptors for GM-CSF. Indeed, receptor numbers are elevated compared with those of litter-mate control peritoneal macrophages.

The diseases exhibited by these transgenic mice raise two questions of importance. First, are the transgenic macrophages activated by internal stimulation by transgenic GM-CSF acting within the cells themselves possibly in an abnormal mode, or are these cells essentially normal and merely showing an extreme physiological response to prolonged stimulation by excess circulating levels of GM-CSF? Second, what mechanisms are responsible for the fibrosis and tissue destruction evident in transgenic mice?

The question of external versus internal GM-CSF stimulation is one with major practical implications. If the response is simply due to excess circulating GM-CSF levels acting on essentially normal cells, then potentially there is a risk in all patients injected with GM-CSF for prolonged periods that a similar sequence of lesions could develop. If, on the other hand, a key requirement is the deranged action of GM-CSF within responding cells, no such risk exists. This question is in urgent need of resolution because, cell for cell, peritoneal macrophages in mice injected with GM-CSF resemble those in transgenic mice.

At this time there is no definitive information on the cellular processes resulting in the fibrotic, inflammatory, or tissue-destructive lesions developing in these mice. However, the most prominent cells present in abnormal numbers and physiological state are the enlarged macrophages. Macrophages have been implicated in the development of arteriosclerotic and other fibrotic lesions because of their ability to produce a variety of molecules including platelet-derived growth factor, fibroblast growth factor, interleukin 1, and tumor necrosis factor. Production by macrophages of at least some of these molecules has been shown to be stimulated by CSF, and therefore a likely explanation for the lesions developing in transgenic mice is that they represent the cellular consequences of CSF stimulation of macrophages.

Evidence that excess CSF production by nonhemopoietic tissues in transgenic mice may not be of great relevance in the genesis of the lesions in these mice has come from observations on the effects of injecting irradiated mice with hemopoietic cells infected in vitro with a retroviral construct containing the GM-CSF gene. Such mice develop very high serum GM-CSF levels, similar muscle lesions, some cellular infiltration of the eye, elevated levels of peritoneal macrophages, and profound macrophage and granulocytic infiltrates in the liver, lungs, lymphoid organs, and heart. The same questions arise concerning the relative roles of high circulating GM-CSF levels versus intracellular expression of GM-CSF in the responding macrophages and granulocytes, but in these mice, excess production of GM-CSF by other tissues can probably be excluded.

Again the speed of development of lesions (within a few weeks) is impressive and has possible implications for patients receiving CSF injections for similar periods.

Summary

The lethal consequences of overexpression of GM-CSF in transgenic mice provide a clear warning that, as is true for all biologically active agents, excess levels of CSF may have long-term damaging effects on tissues. In the case of GM-CSF in the mouse, these effects seem to involve products of activated macrophages, but future studies using G-CSF may reveal toxic effects attributable to materials released from activated polymorphs.

The present observations certainly indicate the need for caution in the clinical use of the CSFs, but, on the positive side, transgenic GM-CSF mice appear to provide fascinating models for the development of some poorly understood disease states. The muscular lesions are similar in nature to those in rheumatic fever, and similar fibrotic lesions occur in man. There have been implications of a role of chronic sepsis or tissue irritation in the development of these conditions, and these are exactly the situations in which chronic overproduction of CSFs might be anticipated. It may be, therefore, that transgenic CSF mice will be able to provide a more complete explanation of the pathogenesis of these puzzling disease states.

10

Role of the CSFs in Myeloid Leukemia

Myeloid leukemia is a clonal neoplasm involving a progressive expansion of granulocyte and monocyte populations with evidence of maturation arrest or abnormal maturation. The location in the hemopoietic hierarchy of the clonogenic cell that initiates what is recognized clinically as myeloid leukemia can vary. As a consequence, other lineages can be members of the leukemic clone. This is most clearly apparent in chronic myeloid leukemia (CML), where the initiating cell must be a member of the stem cell compartment since erythroid cells, eosinophils, megakaryocytes, mast cells, and occasionally B-lymphocytes are also members of the CML clone. The situation is less clear for patients with acute myeloid leukemia (AML). In cases where the disease follows an initial myelodysplastic disorder such as refractory anemia, there is evidence for multilineage involvement comparable with that found in CML. In most AML patients, however, it seems possible that the initiating cell may actually be a granulocyte-macrophage progenitor cell and that the abnormal clone is restricted to this population.

Even though the CSFs, particularly Multi-CSF and GM-CSF, are active on multipotential and stem cells, it may be a serious oversimplification to regard the myeloid leukemias merely as neoplasms of CSF-dependent populations. Nevertheless, because the CSFs are the only known proliferative stimuli for these populations and because the granulocyte-macrophage and related CSF-dependent populations constitute a major component in neoplastic AML and CML populations, it is relevant to consider the role played by the CSFs in the initiation and progression of these diseases.

Autocrine Concepts of Carcinogenesis

The theoretical basis for considering the role of proliferative stimuli in the initiation and emergence of cancers has multiple origins. In the earliest speculations concerning the possible nature of the disorders leading to the autonomous proliferation of a cancer population, one explanation advanced was that the cancer cells might either have become refractory to control by normal regulators or might in fact be producing their own growth factors. In the absence of any knowledge at that time concerning such specific growth factors, this speculation was quite hypothetical.

A major advance in these concepts followed the demonstration by Furth and his colleagues in the early 1950s that in target tissues of classical hormones, cancers could develop if prolonged perturbations were induced in the relative levels of stimulating versus inhibiting hormones. Two distinct phases were noted in such emerging cancers. In the initial phase, the affected cells continued to behave as cancer cells only if the perturbed balance of regulatory hormones was maintained (dependent tumors). Such tumors disappeared following correction of the hormonal imbalance. With time, mutant populations emerged, and these continued to exhibit progressive proliferation even in the absence of hormonal imbalance (autonomous tumors). This change was usually associated with chromosomal abnormalities, loss of specialized functions of the cells, and progressive anaplasia of the tumor tissue.

With the identification in the last decade of tissue-specific growth factors, it was demonstrated that many tumors produce normal or abnormal growth factors able to stimulate the proliferation of cells of the same population. This led to the proposition that cancer cells arise following acquisition by the cells of a capacity to synthesize their own growth factors. In its simplest form, this hypothesis envisaged secretion by a cell of the relevant growth factor, followed by binding of the factor to membrane receptors, thus inducing proliferation (autocrine growth hypothesis). Variants of this hypothesis envisaged that the growth factor might on occasion travel some distance to act on tumor cells (paracrine growth) or function as a humoral regulator throughout the body (exocrine growth). The factors concerned might be structurally normal growth factors or abnormal versions of these molecules.

Work with HTLV 1–induced T-lymphomas introduced an additional possibility: that a cell could become autostimulatory not by growth factor production, but by the synthesis and display of abnormal or abnormally large numbers of growth receptors (in the case of the T-cell leukemias, receptors for the T-cell regulator IL-2).

A number of observations on viral oncogenes and/or their corresponding cellular proto-oncogenes and on chromosomal translocations involving these genes lend general support to the proposition that cancer development is associated with the perturbed formation either of growth factors or of growth factor receptors: (1) *c-sis* encodes the β chain of platelet-derived growth factor; (2) *v-erbB* encodes for a truncated form of the EGF receptor; (3) *c-fms* encodes for the M-CSF receptor; and (4) tumor growth factor (TGFα) has significant homology with epidermal growth factor (EGF) and binds to EGF receptors.

Although there is increasing evidence for disordered growth factor production and/or receptor expression by cancer cells, there are a number of problems associated with this simple explanation of the nature of cancer.

1. Most cancers are clones derived from a single initiating cell. It is difficult to conceive how the first neoplastic cell is able to synthesize sufficiently high amounts of its own growth factor to generate a significant concentration of the factor around the cell and thereby to achieve an adequate level of receptor binding sufficient to activate the cell. This problem is compounded when the cell is located in a moving fluid milieu.

2. In the case of growth factors like the CSFs, there are multiple normal tissue sources of the factor and significant concentrations of the factors preexisting in the serum. Any additional contribution from the first emerging cancer cell would be quite trivial under these conditions.

3. The major deficiency of the simple autocrine concept is that it fails to account for the essential prerequisite of a cancer cell, which is its capacity for an abnormal level of self-generative divisions. In any actively proliferating normal population that maintains a stable size, the number of progeny resembling the parent cell must not exceed 50 percent of the total; otherwise the population increases in size progressively. A normal proliferating population maintains size stability by ensuring equality in the number of parental or differentiative progeny being generated. Under conditions requiring regeneration the balance can be perturbed in favor of self-generation, but on restoration

of correct total numbers, the system again reverts to equality. Clonogenic cancer cells can be demonstrated to be skewed in their proliferative behavior, forming more than 50 percent parental-type progeny; with some cancer cell lines, the proportion can approximate 100 percent. This denotes an intrinsic abnormality in the genetic programing of the cell that is a quite separate issue from the level or source of growth factors impinging on the cell.

Abnormally high stimulation of a cell by either extrinsic or autocrine molecules cannot alone result in a neoplastic pattern of proliferative response, and thus the vital abnormality acquired by cancer cells is that which determines the abnormal pattern of proliferative response following signaling. Studies on immortalized hemopoietic cell lines that are dependent on CSF for survival and proliferation show that the clonogenic cells in the population exhibit an abnormally high capacity for self-generative divisions, yet the cells are not leukemogenic. It is therefore evident that although this anomaly is a necessary property for cancer cells, it is not in itself sufficient to result in a cancer cell.

Alternative Autocrine Models

Leaving aside for the moment the necessity for an intrinsic abnormality in the response of a cancer cell to proliferative signaling, there are a number of alternative mechanisms (Figure 37), all in the general category of autocrine stimulation, that avoid some of the difficulties in the simple concept that autocrine stimulation is achieved by secretion of a growth factor able to stimulate membrane receptors. Each of the alternatives has in fact been demonstrated to occur in various leukemias.

1. Cells may synthesize abnormal numbers or types of membrane receptors that, with or without growth factor binding, are able to elicit the metabolic cascade that normally occurs following binding of a growth factor to its receptor. An example of this is the high IL-2 receptor expression on HTLV-1–transformed T-lymphocytes.

2. Cells may acquire a constitutive capacity to synthesize their own growth factor, but secretion of the molecule is unnecessary, or if it occurs is irrelevant, because effective contact with

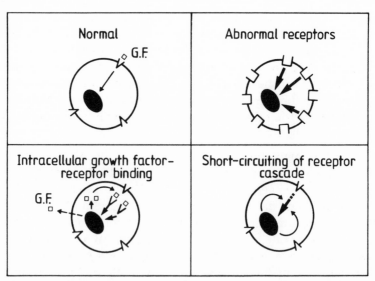

Figure 37. Alternative methods of autostimulation possibly occurring in cancer cells. (*top left*): The conventional process of secretion of a growth factor stimulating the cell via membrane receptors for the growth factor. (*top right*): Autostimulation by abnormal or excessive numbers of receptors. (*lower left*): Autostimulation occurring entirely within the cell, where synthesized growth factor molecules bind to receptor molecules within the cytoplasm. (*lower right*): Autostimulation by abnormal production of a metabolite involved in the signaling pathway normally initiated by binding of the growth factor to its membrane receptor.

receptors is made intracellularly. A likely example of this is the transformation of leukemic FDC-P1 cells by a retrovirus containing the GM-CSF gene (see the section on leukemic transformation of immortalized cell lines later in this chapter).

3. Cells may produce abnormal types or levels of molecules that are a part of the metabolic cascade initiated following binding of growth factors to their membrane receptors. These molecules could activate the remaining sequence of the metabolic cascade and, by so doing, deliver a proliferative signal that bypasses the need for the original signal initiated by binding of growth factor to its receptor. Whether or not such a cell actually secretes a growth factor molecule would be largely irrelevant for the process of self-stimulation. An example of this process is probably the transformation of FDC-P1 cells by the Abelson virus (see the section on leukemic transformation of immortalized cell lines).

Requirements for Involvement of the CSFs in Myeloid Leukemia Development

An analysis of the possible involvement of the CSFs in the initiation and emergence of myeloid leukemic populations needs to consider a number of possibilities: (1) the endocrine tumorigenesis model, where high levels of CSF originating elsewhere in the body place an unbalanced proliferative pressure on granulocytes and macrophages; (2) acquisition by granulocyte-macrophage populations of an ability to synthesize and secrete abnormally high levels of CSF, possibly as a result of chromosomal translocation altering the control sequences operating on the CSF genes; (3) acquisition by granulocyte-macrophage progenitors of an ability to synthesize CSF with wholly internal self-stimulation; (4) acquisition by granulocyte-macrophage precursors of the ability to synthesize key metabolites in the normal cascade elicited by CSF signaling; and (5) expression by granulocyte-macrophage populations of abnormal numbers of CSF receptors able to initiate signaling without the necessity of CSF binding. In all situations it should be demonstrable that the leukemic cells exhibit as a minimum abnormality an abnormal capacity for self-generative divisions, whatever the mode of CSF-related proliferative signaling.

The general alternative to these CSF-related transformations is to postulate that CSFs have no involvement in myeloid leukemic transformation and that such transformation frees the affected cell entirely from its previous dependency on CSF, with proliferation now requiring no specific stimulatory mechanism or being achieved by some quite novel pathway.

Proliferative Behavior of CML and AML Cells In Vitro

The original data from the culture in semisolid medium of leukemic cells from patients with CML or AML appeared to provide quite unambiguous evidence that primary myeloid leukemic cells usually exhibit a continuing absolute dependency on extrinsic CSF for all proliferative activity.

Cells from the marrow or blood of patients with CML proliferate readily in semisolid cultures, forming abnormally large numbers of granulocyte-macrophage colonies. These are identifiable as members of the leukemic clone by their Ph^1 marker. The colonies are of normal size and contain differentiating granulocytes and macrophages. CML clonogenic cells are often of abnormally light, buoyant density and are relatively resistant to inhibition by prostaglandin E, but the colonies generated cannot be distinguished on morphological analysis from normal colonies. This clonogenic proliferation is absolutely dependent on addition to the cultures of adequate concentrations of GM-CSF or G-CSF, the quantitative responsiveness of the cells being indistinguishable from that of normal clonogenic cells. No unstimulated cell proliferation occurs unless crowded cultures are used; in such cases it can be shown that the CSF is generated within the culture dish by monocytes and possibly other adherent cells in the cultured cell population, a phenomenon seen also in cultures of normal cells.

Thus although one mature cell type of the leukemic clone, the monocyte, can undoubtedly produce CSF, this in itself is not abnormal since normal monocytes produce similar levels of CSF and cultures of purified CML clonogenic cells exhibit no capacity for unstimulated proliferation.

Essentially similar conclusions can be drawn from the proliferative behavior of AML cells in culture. Here the proliferative pattern exhibited is quite abnormal; few or no colony-forming cells are present, and the clonogenic leukemic cells generate clusters of varying size often with very low plating efficiency and usually with evidence of abnormal maturation. The poor proliferative capacity exhibited by AML cells in vitro remains puzzling, but, leaving aside this anomaly, cells from the vast majority of patients exhibit a similar absolute dependency on extrinsic GM-CSF or G-CSF to that seen with CML cells (Figure 38). Again their quantitative responsiveness is similar to that of normal GM progenitors, and there is little evidence that individual populations are selectively responsive only to GM-CSF or G-CSF. A few patients have been described whose cells exhibit autonomous proliferation in semisolid cultures under stringent culture conditions, and these do appear to be genuine examples of autocrine self-stimulation since mRNA transcription and CSF synthesis have been demonstrated by the clonogenic cells.

These in vitro observations appeared to eliminate for the vast majority of myeloid leukemic patients the possibility that leukemic transformation resulted from autonomous growth or autoproduction of CSF. However, a formal possibility exists that in vitro culture conditions might be quite misleading in indicating continuing CSF depen-

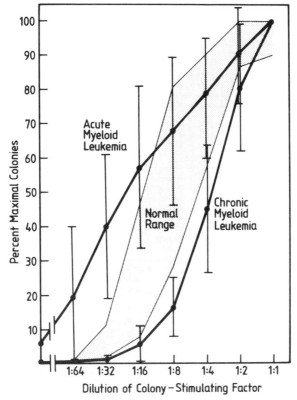

Figure 38. Stimulation by increasing concentrations of CSF of colony formation by normal human marrow cells and leukemic cells from patients with acute or chronic myeloid leukemia. The proliferation seen in some unstimulated cultures of acute myeloid leukemic cells is usually due to CSF production by mature monocytes in the cultured cell population.

dency, and that for some reason the cells are able to behave differently in vivo.

Role of the CSFs in Leukemia Induction

If valid, the in vitro evidence on the continuing dependency of primary human myeloid leukemic cells on CSF indicates that, at the very least, the CSFs must be essential cofactors in the emergence of leukemic populations, since without CSF stimulation the leukemic clone could not proliferate and expand in size.

Since the in vitro data suggest that the leukemic clone is not the major source of CSF, myeloid leukemia development can be considered as one would if analyzing an endocrine tumor induction system. Is there any evidence that low CSF levels prevent myeloid leukemia development, or that high levels either predispose to leukemia development or are present in individuals with myeloid leukemia?

There is no experimental animal with zero CSF production and no method for suppressing CSF levels on a long-term basis. However, the germ-free animal has undetectable circulating CSF levels (even though CSF levels are readily inducible), and it is of interest that whole-body irradiation is unable to induce myeloid leukemia in germ-free mice. Such irradiated mice will develop myeloid leukemia if subsequently conventionalized, a procedure of microbial contamination leading to elevation of circulating CSF levels. These data indirectly support the general thesis that CSF is necessary for the emergence and progressive proliferation of a myeloid leukemic clone.

In about one-third of patients developing AML, the disease is preceded by a myeloproliferative disorder of sufficient severity to attract clinical attention, for example, refractory anemia. Studies of CSF levels in these patients should provide some evidence concerning CSF levels during the last stages of leukemic transformation, especially since only a subset of patients with myeloproliferative disorders actually develops myeloid leukemia. Serum CSF levels have been found to be unremarkable in either subset of patients, but more crucial data would be estimates of CSF levels within the marrow cavity or of the capacity of marrow stromal cells to produce CSF. Data on these parameters are beyond present technical capacity; however, one study observed that a high capacity of adherent marrow cells from myeloproliferative disorder patients to produce CSF was correlated with a low risk of leukemia development. The study was performed before the existence of multiple types of CSF was recognized, and the type of CSF involved is unknown.

In one study on patients with AML or CML, about half of the serum or urine samples exhibited high CSF levels as assayed on mouse bone marrow (and therefore either G-CSF or M-CSF). High CSF levels correlated most strongly with the presence of infections and may therefore merely have been reflecting normal responses to such infections. However, infections are not usually common in CML, and the high CSF levels in these patients could have represented an underlying abnormality in CSF production.

Since marrow stromal cells produce CSF, an indirect method for partially assessing the capacity of marrow cells to produce CSF is to determine the frequency of clonogenic fibroblasts (CFU-F) in marrow populations. In AML marrow samples the frequency of CFU-F is abnormally low in relapse, with levels returning to normal in remission. These data suggest that the production of CSF by some marrow cell types in AML could be subnormal.

Thus the available data on preleukemic and leukemic patients present an inconsistent picture of what levels of CSF may exist, but in general they do not substantiate a simple endocrine tumor induction model in which CSF levels are grossly elevated. The recent development of transgenic GM-CSF mice with constitutively elevated GM-CSF levels may provide a useful model, when extended, for determining the possible leukemogenic effects of high CSF levels.

In view of earlier comments on the necessity for cancer cells to exhibit an intrinsic heritable abnormality in self-generation, it is unlikely that overproduction of CSF either throughout the body or in GM populations themselves could by itself result in myeloid leukemia development. For such overproduction to be effective, an additional event inducing a perturbation in the pattern of proliferation exhibited by the responding GM cells would need to occur.

Leukemic Transformation of CSF-Dependent Immortalized Hemopoietic Cell Lines

It has been possible to develop cloned continuous hemopoietic cell lines from mouse bone marrow, and some of these cell lines exhibit properties of value in analyzing leukemogenesis. Such cell lines, as exemplified by the 32D or FDC-P1 lines, exhibit certain distinctive features. They remain absolutely dependent on CSF for survival and proliferation in vitro. Most lines respond to Multi-CSF, but some are also responsive to GM-CSF, G-CSF, or M-CSF. A high proportion of the cells are clonogenic as assayed in semisolid cultures, and up to 95 percent of the colony cells formed are themselves clonogenic.

The cell lines are thus immortalized and exhibit the high self-renewal trait necessary for neoplastic cells. Despite these characteristics and the presence often of quite marked chromsomal abnormalities, such cell lines are not leukemogenic in normal syngeneic mice.

Because of their properties, these cell lines can be regarded as preleukemic cells, and they can be used in much the same manner as 3T3 cells to explore what additional abnormalities are required to transform the cells to typical leukemic cells. A number of studies of this type have been performed using the FDC-P1 cell line, responsive to stimulation either by GM-CSF or Multi-CSF (Figure 39). The findings are described in the following paragraphs.

1. Insertion into FDC-P1 cells of GM-CSF cDNA in a retroviral construct containing the Moloney virus LTR promoter led to transformation of the cells. The transformed cells proliferated autonomously in semisolid cultures and also were highly leukemogenic in vivo. The cells transcribed high levels of GM-CSF mRNA and secreted large amounts of GM-CSF. Somewhat surprisingly, the cells did not exhibit crowding-dependent proliferation in vitro, as would be expected if secreted CSF were required to bind to membrane receptors to induce proliferation. Furthermore, antiserum against GM-CSF did not inhibit cell proliferation, and the conclusion reached was that even though the cells were clearly secreting large amounts of GM-CSF, the CSF actually being used to self-stimulate the cells was able to act entirely intracytoplasmically. Membrane receptor numbers for GM-CSF remained unaltered, as did the affinity of the receptors.

These experiments indicated that if a cell was already abnormal and possessed high self-renewal capacity, leukemic transformation could be completed simply by inducing the cell to become self-stimulating by producing its own CSF. This provided definitive proof that autocrine CSF production can be a transforming rather than simply a permissive factor, since untransformed FDC-P1 cells are nonleukemic in vivo.

The problem with this model is that the transformed cell lines were clearly autonomous in vitro, unlike naturally occurring primary myeloid leukemic cells from man or the mouse, and thus the model differs radically from the naturally occurring disease.

2. A similar series of transforming experiments using Multi-CSF cDNA also resulted in acquisition by the transformed cells of leukemogenicity, but the behavior of the transformed cells in vitro differed. Some transformed cell lines behaved in an unambiguously autonomous manner similar to those transformed by GM-CSF. However, many of the cloned lines contained a mixture of cells, some being autonomous and others remaining Multi-CSF-dependent. Analysis showed that individual autonomous cells generated progeny most of which were dependent; the molecular basis for this appeared to be a shutdown of mRNA transcription. The dependent cells derived from such autonomous cells remained leukemogenic, al-

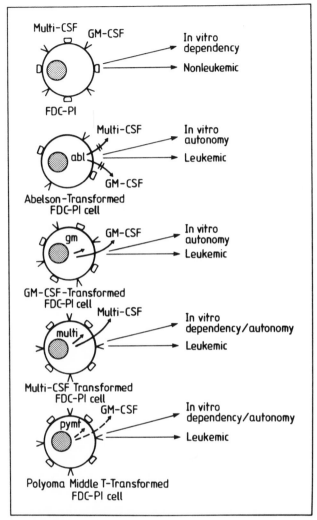

Figure 39. Leukemic transformation of cells of the immortalized cell line FDC-P1 can be achieved by (1) infection with Abelson virus, a process involving neither CSF synthesis nor abnormal CSF receptors; (2) infection with a retrovirus containing GM-CSF cDNA, a process leading to intracytoplasmic stimulation by GM-CSF and the incidental secretion of GM-CSF; (3) infection with a retrovirus containing Multi-CSF cDNA, leading to a similar process; or (4) infection with a retrovirus containing polyoma middle-T cDNA, where possibly intracytoplasmic synthesis and action of GM-CSF again constitute the transforming event. Cells transformed by the latter two methods can sometimes remain CSF-dependent in vitro.

though the latent period to tumor development was longer than with autonomous cells, and the leukemias resulting were not derived from autonomous variants since the cells remained partially CSF-dependent when recultured in vitro. Some transformed cell lines remained fully dependent on extrinsic CSF for survival and proliferation in vitro, but again some of these proved to be leukemogenic in vivo. In contrast to the GM-CSF model, the behavior of dependent Multi-CSF-transformed cells did resemble that of primary human myeloid leukemias in vitro.

These observations on cells whose transformation was achieved simply by inserting an abnormally regulated Multi-CSF gene confirmed the previous observations that acquired self-stimulation could be a transforming event, and again the evidence indicated that the key stimulation occurred intracellularly. However, they introduced a disturbing new possibility: that self-stimulating cells might not necessarily be detectable using clonal in vitro cultures, since the transformed dependent sublines could only reasonably have been transformed by insertion of the Multi-CSF gene yet the cells appeared to remain wholly dependent in vitro on extrinsic CSF. Thus it was possible that a leukemic cell might indeed be able to be self-stimulating in vivo, but with such low levels of transcription and translation that the process would not be detectable by conventional in vitro assays.

Extension of this conclusion to the apparently unambiguous data from the culture of human myeloid leukemic cells raises the possibility that no secure conclusion may be able to be drawn from the apparently dependent behavior of the human leukemic cells in vitro. When one adds to this possibility the evidence that occasional AML populations are clearly capable of autocrine CSF production and self-stimulation and that translocations in leukemic cells commonly involve the CSF gene cluster on chromosome 5 or the G-CSF gene on chromosome 17, the possibility emerges that a far higher proportion of human myeloid leukemias than formerly expected might in fact be engaging in a low but quite crucial level of autoproduction of CSF as a consequence of translocational derangement of control genes. In this type of situation, the autoproduction of even low levels of CSF might lead to transformation even if the CSF remained entirely intracytoplasmic in location.

3. Other studies have emphasized that transformation of FDC-P1 cells need not involve either acquired autocrine CSF production or the display of abnormal numbers of CSF receptors. Thus infection of

FDC-P1 cells with Abelson virus transformed the cells to autonomous leukemic cells with no evidence of transcription of CSF mRNA, synthesis of CSF, or expression of abnormal types or numbers of membrane CSF receptors.

4. Transformation of FDC-P1 cells could be achieved also by infection with a retroviral construct containing the cDNA for polyoma middle-T antigen. The cells episodically produced low levels of GM-CSF, and again different transformed cloned cell lines, all of which were leukemogenic, showed widely differing culture patterns in vitro that did not correlate with their capacity to produce GM-CSF. Some lines were autonomous; some were dependent at all cell concentrations used; others exhibited density-dependent proliferation, suggesting that cell proliferation might be dependent on secretion of low levels of GM-CSF that needed to activate the cells by binding to membrane receptors. The data again emphasized the potential unreliability of in vitro cloning data as a screening procedure to detect autostimulating cells.

In both of the last two examples, it is conceivable that the actual transformation process involved the generation by the *abl* translation product or polyoma middle-T antigen of metabolic intermediates in the signaling pathway usually initiated by binding of CSF to membrane receptors, short-circuiting the full signaling pathway but achieving the same final result of self-stimulation.

In chicken cells where transformation to monocytic leukemia was achieved by sequential infection with *v-myc* and then *v-mil*, the transformed cells secreted M-CSF, and the autonomous proliferation of the transformed cells could be partially blocked by addition of antibodies to the CSF. Here viral transformation may have activated CSF secretion as the mediator of the leukemic transformation rather than merely activating intermediates in the CSF signaling pathway.

Although these studies all involved a quite abnormal starting population with preexisting and probably essential abnormalities in the programing of cellular responses to CSF stimulation, they indicated two important principles: first, that autocrine production of CSF can serve as a final transforming event in leukemia development, and second, that the existence of this process cannot reliably be excluded by the demonstration of CSF-dependency on clonal culture of the cells in vitro.

As mentioned earlier, there is now increasing evidence for translocation involving CSF genes in myeloproliferative disorders and some types of AML, and it is becoming more likely not only that the CSFs function as necessary cofactors supporting the emergence of transformed leukemic populations, but also that the acquisition of low levels of autocrine CSF production by preleukemic cells may represent a final transforming event in many such populations.

Suppression of Myeloid Leukemic Cells by CSFs

Thus far the CSFs have been considered only as mandatory proliferative stimuli for granulocyte-macrophage populations and therefore as likely to be involved in inducing or sustaining the emergence of myeloid leukemic populations. However, the CSFs have an ability to induce irreversible differentiation commitment in responding normal cells. Since an essential abnormality of a leukemic cell is an abnormal predisposition to self-generate, the CSFs could have a significant suppressive influence on leukemic cells if CSF action led to commitment to differentiation and suppression of self-generation, with or without the production of maturing postmitotic progeny.

Evidence that the CSFs can suppress myeloid leukemic populations has come mainly from studies on the WEHI-3B murine myelomonocytic leukemic model. Cells of this established line exhibit a high level (greater than 90 percent) of self-generative divisions; fail to mature beyond early promyelocytes or promonocytes; have acquired complete autonomy with respect to exogenous CSF in culture; and are highly leukemogenic in vivo. They also constitutively synthesize Multi-CSF, but it is unclear whether this process was relevant to their original transformation. Two major sublines of WEHI-3B exist, the D^+ (capable of differentiation induction) and the D^- (a tetraploid cell line with the morphology of immature macrophages that is refractory to differentiation induction). D^- cells on a per cell basis produce more Multi-CSF than do D^+ cells and the lines differ with respect to membrane CSF receptors, D^+ cells exhibiting receptors for G-CSF while D^- cells do not.

Addition of G-CSF to semisolid cultures of WEHI-3B D^+ cells leads to the formation of colonies that are surrounded by a prominent halo of differentiating monocytes and granulocytes (Figure 40). Some colonies are composed wholly of differentiating cells and are usually small in size. Sequential analysis of colony formation in the presence of G-CSF indicates that initial clonal growth is slightly more rapid than in cultures lacking G-CSF, possibly indicating a residual responsiveness of the cells to proliferative stimulation by G-CSF. As differ-

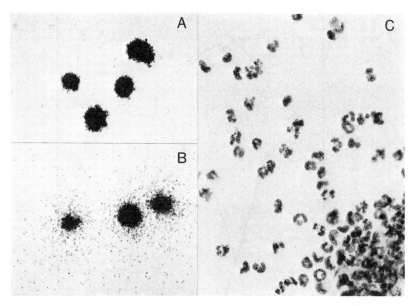

Figure 40. Induction of differentiation in WEHI-3B leukemic colonies by culture in the presence of G-CSF. (*A*) Control WEHI-3B colonies. (*B*) WEHI-3B colonies exhibiting halos of differentiating granulocytes and monocytes induced by G-CSF. (*C*) High-power view of differentiating cells in a leukemic colony grown in the presence of G-CSF.

entiation becomes more prominent, however, the increase in colony size slows, and if all cells differentiate, final colony size can be very small.

The phenomenon is a dramatic example of the ability of a normal regulator molecule to induce differentiation in certified leukemic cells, although the differentiating cells are commonly somewhat abnormal in size, shape, nuclear morphology, and membrane markers.

What is of more significance is the fact that G-CSF induces a pronounced reduction in the level of self-generation by clonogenic WEHI-3B D$^+$ cells; if colony cells are recultured in the presence of G-CSF for two to five culture sequences, the leukemic population becomes devoid of clonogenic cells and the population is extinguished (Figure 41). G-CSF has no capacity to induce differentiation in WEHI-3B D$^-$ cells, if for no other reason than that they lack G-CSF receptors.

GM-CSF also exhibits a capacity to induce differentiation in WEHI-3B cells, but the action is weaker than that of G-CSF and the level of

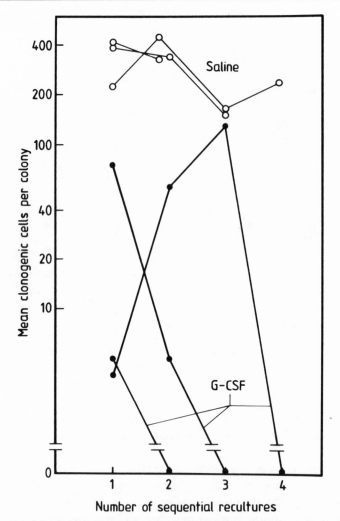

Figure 41. Suppression of clonogenic cells in WEHI-3B colonies by sequential reculture of colony cells in the presence of G-CSF. Despite some initial variability, clonogenic cell formation is eventually suppressed by G-CSF.

suppression of clonogenic self-renewal is insufficient to extinguish the population. M-CSF and Multi-CSF have no differentiation-inducing actions on this leukemia.

Analysis using daughter, granddaughter, and later progeny of individual WEHI-3B cells has shown that the commitment induced by G-CSF is irreversible and is achieved through two stages: (1) induction

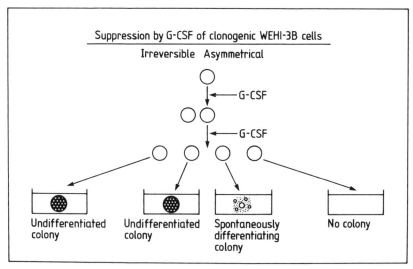

Figure 42. A typical example of changes induced in granddaughter cells of a clonogenic WEHI-3B leukemic cell by culture in the presence of G-CSF. After washing to remove G-CSF, two cells appeared unaltered, one cell formed a spontaneously differentiating colony, and one formed a small clone of differentiated cells that died during the culture period.

in the cells of a capacity to exhibit spontaneous differentiation following removal of the G-CSF, although the cells remain able to generate colonies; and (2) absolute suppression of clonogenicity, the cells sometimes dying but more commonly generating two to four differentiating progeny. Commitment is markedly asymmetrical: typically among four granddaughters, one or two may remain apparently unaltered, one generates a spontaneously differentiating colony, and one is suppressed (Figure 42). Brief exposure of cells to G-CSF for a few hours is insufficient to induce differentiation commitment; the process appears to require passage through one or two cell cyles in the presence of G-CSF. Other studies on differentiation commitment of leukemic cells using chemical inducers such as butyric acid or phorbol esters suggest that the decision point in the cell cycle regarding commitment may be at the G_1-S interface. However, in the G-CSF induction system with its notable asymmetry, commitment events could occur during chromosomal duplication, with the newly synthesized daughter chromatid possibly being particularly prone to methylation or some other irreversible modification.

The concentrations of G-CSF required to induce differentiation in

WEHI-3B cells are identical to those required to stimulate the formation of normal granulocytic colonies by normal bone marrow cells. G-CSF also has differentiation-inducing effects on another murine myeloid leukemic cell line, the M1, but the concentrations required to induce differentiation in this line are higher than for WEHI-3B D^+ cells.

It has been shown that the injection of G-CSF into mice transplanted with WEHI-3B D^+ leukemic cells is capable of suppressing the development of myeloid leukemia and permitting survival of the animals.

These studies indicate that G-CSF, and to a lesser degree GM-CSF, can have powerful suppressive effects on myeloid leukemic populations that override any initial proliferative stimulation. If the results are generally applicable, the role of the CSFs in myeloid leukemia development becomes quite complex: they are seen to be both initiators and suppressors of emerging leukemic clones. It is now necessary to reexamine questions concerning the production and levels of CSFs during leukemogenesis in more detail than previously envisaged, investigating not only overall CSF levels but which particular CSFs are involved.

The situation with human leukemic cells is less clear. G-CSF is an effective proliferative stimulus for most CML and AML populations (Figure 43). There is little evidence of more pronounced differentiation induction in CML colonies stimulated by G-CSF as compared with GM-CSF; in both cases differentiation is complete and colonies contain no clonogenic cells. It has usually been argued that CML clonogenic cells are quite mature and, like normal GM progenitors, have no capacity for self-generation. Now, however, it cannot be excluded that the CSF used to stimulate colony formation has simultaneously suppressed a preexisting capacity for the clonogenic cells for self-renewal. In cultures of AML cells, morphological differentiation is incomplete and usually aberrant. It has been reported that G-CSF is superior to GM-CSF in inducing at least partial differentiation in clonal progeny of AML cells, but again a problem exists with such clones because they usually contain no clonogenic cells, whether as a result of the nature of the cells or of CSF action.

Blast colony formation by AML leukemic cells is probably due to the proliferation of more ancestral stem cells in the population since the blast colonies contain cells with some, if limited, capacity for recloning. However, combined use of GM-CSF and G-CSF resulted in

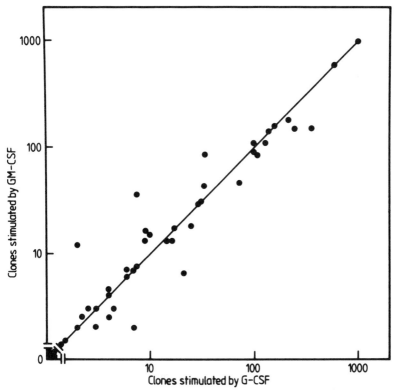

Figure 43. Comparison of the proliferative effects of GM-CSF and G-CSF in clonal cultures of primary human acute myeloid leukemic cells. Cells from most patients responded equally to proliferative stimulation by both CSFs despite the wide differences in cloning efficiency seen with cells from different patients. In only one instance were the leukemic cells able to proliferate in the absence of CSF.

larger and more numerous blast cell colonies than with GM-CSF alone, providing little evidence for a suppressive action of G-CSF.

It is also a matter of some concern that although all AML populations (except possibly M5 AMLs) contain cells with receptors for G-CSF, autoradiographic studies indicate that a significant subset of blast cells in any one population lacks G-CSF receptors. This might indicate that G-CSF would be unable to suppress such a population because, in the presence of G-CSF, the population could be over-grown by cells lacking G-CSF receptors. This situation is not true for acute promyelocytic leukemia populations because all cells express

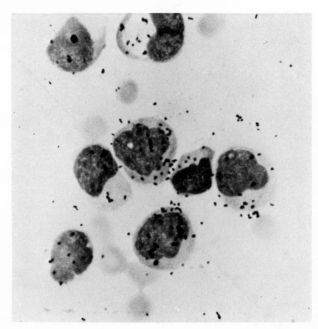

Figure 44. Autoradiograph of acute promyelocytic leukemic cells binding ^{125}I-labeled G-CSF and showing uniform levels of receptors.

large numbers of G-CSF receptors (Figure 44), and leukemic cells of this type seem more likely candidates for suppression by G-CSF.

There are few satisfactory human leukemic cell lines available for testing in the manner used for the murine WEHI-3B leukemia. However, studies using GM-CSF and G-CSF on the HL60 line have indicated that continuous culture of the cells in the presence of CSF can reduce clonogenic self-renewal, and again the phenomenon was more evident with G-CSF than GM-CSF. A feature of these responses was the lack of morphological differentiation in the population being suppressed, although the cells did express enhanced levels of membrane markers characteristic of differentiating cells. It is evident, therefore, that suppression of clonogenic self-renewal does not necessarily need to be accompanied by overt morphological differentiation.

The suppressive effects, particularly of G-CSF, on at least some model myeloid leukemias raise two points of interest, one theoretical and the other practical. First, the abnormal level of self-generation exhibited by leukemic stem cells seems not to be an irreversible characteristic but to be subject to profound modification by the action of extrinsic regulatory molecules. Extension of this principle to other types of cancer raises the possibility that, with appropriate regulator molecules, it may be possible to suppress a wide range of cancer populations.

A similar conclusion can be reached from the competitive behavior between leukemic and normal cells in vivo versus in vitro. In vivo in AML, the leukemic clone dominates and completely suppresses preexisting normal granulocyte-macrophage progenitors. In CML the normal progenitors do not seem to be depressed, but they become vastly outnumbered by the dominant Ph[1] clone. In long-term in vitro cultures, the opposite situation exists: AML and often CML populations decline in such cultures with the reemergence and dominance of normal populations. Again the data suggest the reversibility of the high self-renewal characteristics of leukemic stem cells and the potential for normal cells to compete effectively with leukemic cells, given changes in microenvironmental and/or humoral regulatory control.

One type of differentiation-unresponsive state resulting from the absence of membrane receptors for G-CSF was noted earlier. However, there are other myeloid and myelomonocytic leukemias that do express membrane receptors for G-CSF yet are equally refractory to either suppression or differentiation induction by G-CSF. In such populations it is likely that abnormal genetic programing no longer permits a response to G-CSF-initiated signaling. What is intriguing in this context is a number of reports that preexposure of refractory cells to a variety of chemical agents, including cytotoxic drugs used in the treatment of AML, induces a responsive state to differentiation induction. The mechanisms involved have not been studied and are in urgent need of examination. The possibility exists that cytotoxic drugs induce remissions in AML not merely by cytotoxic action but by inducing responsiveness to differentiation induction, a process that could account much better for prolonged remissions lasting several years than speculations about the number of surviving unaltered cells following cytotoxic reduction of leukemic population size. If indeed the action of cytotoxic drugs is far more complex than previously envisaged, the biological significance of differentiation induction by regulatory molecules becomes of greater importance.

The second point is that the current availability of recombinant human GM-CSF and G-CSF raises the possibility that these agents could be used in the direct suppression of leukemic populations. There is a clear risk involved in such an approach because the same molecules are growth-stimulatory. Nevertheless, if the WEHI-3B D[+] model is a valid one, the suppressive effects of G-CSF can outstrip any initial growth-stimulating effects. The prospects for the use of CSFs combined with chemotherapy seem best for the acute promyelocytic leukemias, which have been noted for their dramatic response to chemotherapy, their more uniform differentiation, and their high levels of expression of membrane receptors for G-CSF. For these reasons, these would seem to be the most appropriate leukemias to treat by a very cautious addition of G-CSF to existing therapy. The same arguments apply to the use of CSFs to accelerate the regeneration of normal hemopoietic tissue following marrow transplantation in AML if some residual leukemic cells persist. There is a distinct risk involved in the use of CSFs to promote regeneration under these conditions, and again G-CSF would seem to be the safest agent for careful trials restricted initially to acute promyelocytic patients.

Summary

The CSFs play a central role in the biology of acute and chronic myeloid leukemia. Myeloid leukemic cells remain dependent on the CSFs for proliferative stimulation, and thus the latter are essential cofactors in the emergence of myeloid leukemias. In some leukemogenesis studies their role seems to extend further than this in that acquired autosynthesis of CSF is a necessary event in the actual process of leukemic transformation. However, attempts at therapy based on suppression of CSF levels are not feasible because surviving normal granulocyte-macrophage populations require CSF for proliferation, and without such populations the patient is defenseless against infections. Paradoxically, at least in some myeloid leukemias, the differentiation commitment action of the CSFs, seen most clearly with G-CSF, can result in effective suppression of myeloid leukemic clones without a comparable action on normal populations, since new progenitor cells are generated continuously from stem cells.

The CSFs are not the only biological agents able to suppress myeloid leukemic populations by inhibitory or differentiation-inducing actions. Differentiation-inducing or leukemia-inhibitory factors (DIF, LIF) have been purified from both human and murine tissues. The human factor appears to be tumor necrosis factor (TNFα), but this is not the case for the murine factor. It is unclear at present how important DIF, LIF, or TNFα may be in vivo and whether they play any role in the control of normal hemopoietic populations. What can be said is that these molecules represent additional agents for possible use in the control of myeloid leukemic populations by biological methods, and that their existence emphasizes the complexity of events occurring during leukemia development.

Myeloid leukemias need not of necessity arise as a consequence of deranged autosynthesis of CSF, but for those that do, the varying biological effects of the different CSFs can lead to a highly complex, competitive situation of promotion versus suppression. Much more information is needed from in vitro studies on the likely outcome of such competitive interactions before decisions can be made regarding the potential of the CSFs as nontoxic therapeutic agents in myeloid leukemia.

The myeloid leukemias can now be added to the tumors of endocrine target tissues as examples of cancers of which the course is not necessarily irreversible but which can be arrested or suppressed by the action of normal regulatory molecules. Such actions cannot reverse preexisting intrinsic abnormalities in cancer cells, but they may slow or prevent the acquisition of further abnormalities in the cells and can certainly arrest the progressive expansion of the tumor population.

Coming at a time when it is becoming recognized that there are limits to what can be achieved by the cytotoxic therapy of cancers, the work on the myeloid leukemias suggests the value of extending this approach to the control of a wide variety of other cancers.

Conclusion

The discovery and characterization of the glycoprotein colony-stimulating factors have allowed a detailed picture to be built up concerning the positive control of granulocyte-macrophage production and some aspects of the functional activation of these cells. The populations of progenitor cells and their progeny that are regulated by the CSFs are of course transit populations generated by more ancestral stem cells, and a proper understanding of the biology of these populations ultimately requires a much more complete knowledge of the manner in which stem cell populations are regulated and in particular of the role played by specialized stromal cells in these processes. There are many aspects of the action of the CSFs that require further clarification; relatively little is known of specific inhibitory or modulating factors that can be presumed to exist and that form an important component of a balanced regulatory system.

Even from what is already known, the CSFs present a number of novel biological features, many of which are likely to hold true also for specific regulators of other cell types. The most closely related regulators are those for other hemopoietic populations. For most of these, information on their detailed actions is less complete than for the CSFs, but similar patterns are emerging. The regulators of other hemopoietic lineages are also glycoproteins, similar in general nature to the CSFs. Most have clearly demonstrable proliferative actions similar to those of the CSFs, and at comparable concentrations. For some regulators such as IL-5 and IL-1, target cell survival in vitro is factor-dependent as is the case for the CSFs, and it is becoming obvious that, like the CSFs, these molecules also have a capacity to stimulate end cell functional activity. From what is known so far about cellular sources, the common features again emerging are those of multicellular origins, lability of synthesis rates, and responses to a multiplicity of induction signals.

The hemopoietic regulators are members of a growing class of regulatory molecules that are distinctly different from the classical hormones in being multicellular in origin and having a quite restricted range of responding target cells but a multiplicity of actions on such cells. The most interesting single aspect of this new class of hormonal regulators is that they dispel the old notion that regulation of cell proliferation and regulation of functional activity are very different aspects of the biology of cells, likely to be controlled by quite different regulators.

Even though there are special reasons why humoral regulators need to be used in the control of hemopoietic populations, there is also evidence that part of the control of hemopoiesis is by cell contact processes. What is emerging is evidence that these two types of regulatory actions may be employing similar molecules, and that the apparent difference may simply be a question of secreted versus membrane-displayed molecules of the same type.

What lessons does this information have for the control of cell populations in solid or stratified tissues such as the liver, gut, or skin? Superficially, the control of such tissues might be expected to be cell contact–based, yet the same requirements need to be met for these tissues as were apparent for hemopoietic tissues. The body needs a minimum number of cells of each type for survival, and some method must exist for determining how many of each particular cell type are present, where they are located, and what differentiation status they have achieved. The same demand-supply rules seem to be applicable as in the case of hemopoietic cells.

It is therefore not improbable that circulating specific regulators exist for liver, gut, and skin populations that are comparable in nature and function to the hemopoietic regulators, even though it is possible that the display of such molecules on adjacent cells may be a more important process than for hemopoietic populations. The prospects of being able to detect such regulators seem good and will be restricted only by the availability of adequate in vitro cell assays able to exhibit measurable responses to such factors. The existence of suitable in vitro bioassay systems was the key to success for the detection of the hemopoietic regulators and is clearly the necessary technology to develop for other cell types. In retrospect, much of the detection of hemopoietic regulators could have been achieved by the judicious use of appropriate leukemic or continuous cell lines. If it is currently difficult to develop satisfactory clonal primary cultures of normal liver or gut cells, then an alternative is to use a variety of tumor populations derived from such cells, naturally treating the data with some caution because of the use of abnormal cells.

What has emerged from the last few years with the entry of molecular biology into the hemopoietic regulator field is that it may no longer be necessary to engage in the tedious process of purifying native regulatory molecules. A more rapid possible alternative is the direct screening of cDNA libraries for such regulatory molecules, although success in this approach also requires adequate in vitro assay systems. An even more radical alternative is the use of transgenic mice to establish the function and role of a candidate polypeptide product, an approach that, while labor-intensive, bypasses all the in vitro steps in the investigation. Although transgenic mice seem likely to become of increasing importance in the future, some initial indirect or in vitro evidence will still be necessary to select candidate cDNA or genomic clones likely to be coding for relevant molecules, if for no other reason than to reduce the labor involved.

The multiple nature of the CSFs concerned with the regulation of granulocytes and macrophages emphasizes a principle familiar to physiologists, namely that multiple control systems operate on all organ and cellular activities. There are obvious evolutionary advantages in the use of such overlapping systems, but the situation certainly presents formidable difficulties when one attempts to define in complete form the regulation of any cell system, including hemopoietic populations.

For those working for the past twenty years on the colony-stimulating factors, it has been a matter of some satisfaction to witness the story unfolding from incidental observation to clinical evaluation of agents that have bright prospects of being significant factors in the management of life-threatening illnesses.

Suggested Readings / Credits / Index

Suggested Readings

1. The Basic Biology of Hemopoiesis

Bradley, T. R., and D. Metcalf. 1966. The growth of mouse bone marrow cells in vitro. *Aust. J. Exp. Biol. Med. Sci.* 44:287–300.

Dieterlen-Lievre, F. 1982. The segregation of intraembryonic blood stem cells during avian development. In *Expression of Differentiated Functions in Cancer Cells*, ed. R. P. Revotella, G. M. Pontieri, S. Basilico, G. Rovera, R. C. Gallo, and J. H. Subak-Sharpe. New York: Raven Press, pp. 1–14.

Goldschneider, I., D. Metcalf, F. Battye, and T. Mandel. 1980. Analysis of rat hemopoietic cells on the fluorescence-activated cell sorter: I. Isolation of pluripotent hemopoietic stem cells and granulocyte-macrophage progenitor cells. *J. Exp. Med.* 152:419–437.

Ichikawa, Y., D. H. Pluznik, and L. Sachs. 1966. In vitro control of the development of macrophage and granulocyte colonies. *Proc. Natl. Acad. Sci. (USA)* 56:488–495.

Metcalf, D. 1984. *Hemopoietic Colony Stimulating Factors.* Amsterdam: Elsevier.

Metcalf, D., and M. A. S. Moore. 1971. *Haemopoietic Cells.* Amsterdam: North-Holland.

Nicola, N. A., A. W. Burgess, F. G. Staber, G. R. Johnson, D. Metcalf, and F. Battye. 1980. Differential expression of lectin receptors during hemopoietic differentiation: Enrichment for granulocyte-macrophage progenitor cells. *J. Cell. Physiol.* 103:217–237.

Pluznik, D. H., and L. Sachs. 1965. The cloning of normal "mast" cells in tissue cultures. *J. Cell. Comp. Physiol.* 66:319–324.

Suda, J., T. Suda, and M. Ogawa. 1984. Analysis of differentiation of mouse hemopoietic stem cells in culture by sequential replating of paired progenitors. *Blood* 64:393–399.

Till, J. E., and E. A. McCulloch. 1961. A direct measurement of the radiation sensitivity of normal mouse bone marrow cells. *Radiat. Res.* 14:213–222.

2. General Aspects of the Control of Hemopoiesis

Dexter, T. M., T. D. Allen, and L. G. Lajtha. 1977. Conditions controlling the proliferation of haemopoietic stem cells in vitro. *J. Cell. Physiol.* 91:335–344.

Dexter, T. M., F. Spooncer, P. Simmons, and T. D. Allen. 1984. Long-term marrow culture: An overview of techniques and experience. In *Long-Term Bone Marrow Cultures*, ed. D. G. Wright and J. S. Greenberger. New York: Alan R. Liss, Kroc Foundation Series, vol. 18:57–96.

Johnson, G. R., and D. Metcalf. 1979. The commitment of multipotential hemopoietic stem cells: Studies in vivo and in vitro. In *Cell Lineage, Stem Cells and Cell Determination*, INSERM Symposium no. 10, ed. N. Le Douarin, Amsterdam: Elsevier/North-Holland, pp. 199–213.

Wolf, N. S. 1979. The haemopoietic microenvironment. *Clin. Haematol.* 8:469–500.

Zipori, D. 1986. Cultured stromal cell lines from hemopoietic tissues. In *Blood Cell Formation: The Role of the Hemopoietic Microenvironment*, ed. M. Tavassoli. New York: Marcel Dekker.

3. The Colony-Stimulating Factors and Their Receptors

Burgess, A. W., J. Camakaris, and D. Metcalf. 1977. Purification and properties of colony-stimulating factor from mouse lung conditioned medium. *J. Biol. Chem.* 252:1998–2003.

Clark, S. C., and R. Kamen. 1987. The human hematopoietic colony-stimulating factors. *Science* 236:1229–1237.

Fung, M. C., A. J. Hapel, S. Ymer, D. R. Cohen, R. M. Johnson, H. D. Campbell, and I. G. Young. Molecular cloning of cDNA for murine interleukin-3. *Nature* 307:233–237.

Gasson, J. C., R. H. Weisbart, S. E. Kaufman, S. C. Clark, R. M. Hewick, and G. G. Wong. 1984. Purified human granulocyte-macrophage colony-stimulating factor: Direct actions on neutrophils. *Science* 226:1339–1342.

Gough, N. M., J. Gough, D. Metcalf, A. Kelso, D. Grail, N. A. Nicola, A. W. Burgess, and A. R. Dunn. 1984. Molecular cloning of cDNA encoding a murine haematopoietic growth regulator, granulocyte-macrophage colony stimulating factor. *Nature* 309:763–767.

Ihle, J. N., J. Keller, L. Henderson, F. Klein, and E. Palaszynski. 1982. Procedures for the purification of interleukin 3 to homogeneity. *J. Immunol.* 129:2431–2436.

Kawasaki, E. S., M. B. Ladner, A. M. Wang, J. Van Arsdell, M. K. Warren, M. Y. Coyne, V. L. Schweickart, M-T. Lee, K. J. Wilson, A. Boosman, E. R. Stanley, P. Ralph, and D. F. Mark. 1985. Molecular cloning of a complementary DNA encoding human macrophage-specific colony-stimulating factor (CSF-1). *Science* 230:291–296.

Metcalf, D. 1984. *The Hemopoietic Colony Stimulating Factors.* Amsterdam: Elsevier.

Nagata, S., M. Tsuchiya, S. Asano, Y. Kaziro, T. Yamazaki, O. Yamamoto, Y. Hirata, N. Kubota, M. Oheda, H. Nomura, and M. Ono. 1986. Molecular cloning and expression of cDNA for human granulocyte-stimulating factor. *Nature* 319:415–418.

Nicola, N. A. 1987. Why do hemopoietic growth factor receptors interact with each other? *Immunology Today* 8:134–140.

Nicola, N. A., D. Metcalf, M. Matsumoto, and G. R. Johnson. 1983. Purification of a factor inducing differentiation in murine myelomonocytic leukemia cells: Identification as granulocyte colony-stimulating factor (G-CSF). *J. Biol. Chem.* 258:9017–9023.

Sherr, C. J., C. W. Rettermier, R. Sacca, M. F. Roussel, A. T. Look, and E. R. Stanley. 1985. The c-fms protooncogene product is related to the receptor for the mononuclear phagocyte growth factor, CSF-1. *Cell* 41:665–676.

Souza, L. M., T. C. Boone, J. Gabrilove, P. H. Lai, K. M. Zebo, D. C. Murdoch, V. R. Chazen, J. Bruszewski, H. Lu, K. K. Chen, J. Barendt, E. Platzer, M. A. S. Moore, R. Mertelsmann, and K. Welte. 1986. Recombinant human granulocyte colony-stimulating factor: Effects on normal and leukemic myeloid cells. *Science* 232:61–65.

Stanley, E. R., G. Hansen, J. Woodcock, and D. Metcalf. 1975. Colony stimulating factor and the regulation of granulopoiesis and macrophage production. *Fed. Proc.* 34:2272–2278.

Stanley, E. R., and P. M. Heard. 1977. Factors regulating macrophage production and growth: Purification and some properties of the colony stimulating factor from medium conditioned by mouse L cells. *J. Biol. Chem.* 252:4305–4312.

Walker, F., N. A. Nicola, D. Metcalf, and A. W. Burgess. 1985. Hierarchical down-modulation of hemopoietic growth factor receptors. *Cell* 43:269–276.

Welte, K., E. Platzer, L. Lu, J. L. Gabrilove, E. Levi, R. Mertelsmann, and M. A. S. Moore. 1985. Purification and biochemical characterization of human pluripotent hematopoietic colony-stimulating factor. *Proc. Natl. Acad. Sci. (USA)* 82:1526–1530.

Wong, G. G., J. S. Witek, P. A. Temple, K. M. Wilkens, A. C. Leary, D. P. Luxenberg, S. S. Jones, E. L. Brown, R. M. Kay, E. C. Orr, C. Shoemaker, D. W. Golde, R. J. Kaufman, R. M. Hewick, E. A. Wang, and S. C. Clark. 1985. Human GM-CSF: Molecular cloning of the complementary DNA and purification of the natural and recombinant proteins. *Science* 228:810–815.

Yang, Y.-C., A. B. Ciarletta, P. A. Temple, M. P. Chung, S. Kovacic, J. S. Witek-Giannotti, A. C. Leary, R. Kriz, R. E. Donahue, G. G. Wong, and S. C. Clark. 1986. Human IL-3 (Multi-CSF): Identification by expression cloning of a novel hematopoietic growth factor related to murine IL-3. *Cell* 47:3–10.

Yokota, T., F. Lee, D. Rennick, C. Hall, N. Arai, T. Mosmann, G. Nabel, H. Cantor, and K.-I. Arai. 1984. Isolation and characterization of a mouse cDNA clone that expresses mast cell growth factor activity in monkey cells. *Proc. Natl. Acad. Sci. (USA)* 81:1070–1074.

4. Biological Effects of the CSFs on Hemopoietic Cells In Vitro

Arnaout, M. A., E. A. Wang, S. C. Clark, and C. A. Sieff. 1986. Human recombinant granulocyte-macrophage colony-stimulating factor increases cell to cell adhesion and surface expression of adhesion promoting surface glycoproteins on mature granulocytes. *J. Clin. Invest.* 78:579–601.

Begley, C. G., A. F. Lopez, N. A. Nicola, D. J. Warren, D. Metcalf, and C. J. Sanderson. 1986. Purified colony stimulating factors enhance the survival of human neutrophils and eosinophils in vitro: A rapid and sensitive microassay for colony stimulating factors. *Blood* 68:162–166.

Grabstein, K. H., D. Urdal, R. J. Tushinski, D. Y. Mochizuki, V. L. Price, M. A. Cantrell, S. Gillis, and P. J. Conlon. 1986. Induction of macrophage tumoricidal activity by granulocyte-macrophage colony-stimulating factor. *Science* 232:506–508.

Hamilton, J. A., E. R. Stanley, A. W. Burgess, and R. K. Shadduck. 1980. Stimulation of macrophage plasminogen activator activity by colony-stimulating factors. *J. Cell. Physiol.* 103:435–445.

Handman, E., and A. W. Burgess. 1979. Stimulation by granulocyte-macrophage colony stimulating factor of Leishmania tropica killing by macrophages. *J. Immunol.* 122:1134–1137.

Kurland, J. I., L. M. Pelus, P. Ralph, R. S. Bockman, and M. A. S. Moore. 1979. Induction of prostaglandin E synthesis in normal and neoplastic macrophages: Role for colony-stimulating factor(s) distinct from effects on myeloid progenitor cell proliferation. *Proc. Natl. Acad. Sci. (USA)* 76:2326–2330.

Lopez, A. F., N. A. Nicola, A. W. Burgess, D. Metcalf, F. L. Battye, W. A. Sewell, and M. Vadas. 1983. Activation of granulocyte cytotoxic function by purified mouse colony-stimulating factors. *J. Immunol.* 131:2983–2988.

Metcalf, D. 1980. Clonal analysis of proliferation and differentiation of paired daughter cells: Action of granulocyte-macrophage colony-stimulating factor on granulocyte-macrophage precursors. *Proc. Natl. Acad. Sci. (USA)* 77:5327–5330.

Metcalf, D., C. G. Begley, N. A. Nicola, and G. R. Johnson. 1987. Quantitative responsiveness of murine hemopoietic populations in vitro and in vivo to recombinant Multi-CSF (IL-3). *Exp. Hematol.* 15:288–297.

Metcalf, D., and A. W. Burgess. 1982. Clonal analysis of progenitor cell commitment to granulocyte and macrophage production. *J. Cell. Physiol.* 111:275–284.

Metcalf, D., A. W. Burgess, G. R. Johnson, N. A. Nicola, E. C. Nice, J. DeLamarter, D. R. Thatcher, and J-J. Mermod. 1986. In vitro actions on hemopoietic cells of recombinant murine GM-CSF purified after production in E. coli: Comparison with purified native GM-CSF. *J. Cell. Physiol.* 128:421–431.

Metcalf, D., G. R. Johnson, and A. W. Burgess. 1980. Direct stimulation by purified GM-CSF of the proliferation of multipotential and erythroid precursor cells. *Blood* 55:138–147.

Metcalf, D., and S. Merchav. 1982. Effects of GM-CSF deprivation on precursors of granulocytes and macrophages. *J. Cell. Physiol.* 112:411–418.

Metcalf, D., S. Merchav, and G. Wagemaker. 1982. Commitment by GM-CSF or M-CSF of bipotential GM progenitor cells to granulocyte or macrophage colony formation. In *Experimental Hematology Today 1982*, ed. S. J. Baum, G. D. Ledney, and S. Thierfelder. Basel: Karger, pp. 3–9.

Metcalf, D., and N. A. Nicola. 1983. Proliferative effects of purified granulocyte colony-stimulating factor (G-CSF) on normal mouse hemopoietic cells. *J. Cell. Physiol.* 116:198–206.

Nicola, N. A., and D. Metcalf. 1986. The colony-stimulating factors and myeloid leukaemia. *Cancer Surveys* 4:789–815.

Vadas, M. A., N. A. Nicola, and D. Metcalf. 1983. Activation of antibody-dependent cell-mediated cytotoxicity of human neutrophils and eosinophils by separate colony-stimulating factors. *J. Immunol.* 130: 795–799.

Vadas, M. A., G. Varigos, N. Nicola, S. Pincus, A. Dessein, D. Metcalf, and F. L. Battye. 1983. Eosinophil activation by colony-stimulating factor in man: Metabolic effects and analysis by flow cytometry. *Blood* 61:1232–1242.

Warren, M. K., and P. Ralph. 1986. Macrophage growth factor CSF-1 stimulates human monocyte production of interferon, tumor necrosis factor, and myeloid CSF. *J. Immunol.* 137:2281–2285.

Weisbart, R. H., D. W. Golde, S. C. Clark, G. G. Wong, and J. C. Gasson. 1985. Human granulocyte-macrophage colony-stimulating factor is a neutrophil activator. *Nature* 314:361–363.

Whetton, A. D., and T. M. Dexter. 1985. Effect of haematopoietic cell growth factor on intracellular ATP levels. *Nature* 303:639–631.

5. *Sites and Control of CSF Production and Degradation*

Bagby, G. C., E. McCall, and D. L. Layman. 1983. Regulation of colony stimulating activity production: Interactions of fibroblasts, mononuclear phagocytes and lactoferrin. *J. Clin. Invest.* 71:340–344.

Bartocci, A., J. W. Pollard, and E. R. Stanley. 1986. Regulation of colony stimulating factor 1 during pregnancy. *J. Exp. Med.* 164:956–961.

Johnson, G. R., and D. Metcalf. 1978. Sources and nature of granulocyte-macrophage colony stimulating factor in fetal mice. *Exp. Hematol.* 6:327–335.

Kelso, A., D. Metcalf, and N. M. Gough. 1986. Independent regulation of granulocyte-macrophage colony stimulating factor and multilineage colony stimulating factor production in T lymphocyte clones. *J. Immunol.* 136:1718–1725.

Metcalf, D. 1971. Acute antigen-induced elevation of serum colony stimulating factor (CSF) levels. *Immunology* 21:427–436.

Munker, R., J. Gasson, M. Ogawa, and H. P. Koeffler. 1986. Recombinant human TNF induces production of granulocyte-monocyte colony-stimulating factor. *Nature* 323:79–82.

Sheridan, J. W., and D. Metcalf. 1972. Studies on the bone marrow colony stimulating factor (CSF): Relation of tissue CSF to serum CSF. *J. Cell. Physiol.* 80:129–140.

Sieff, C. A., S. Tsai, and D. V. Faller. 1987. Interleukin-1 induces cultured human endothelial cell production of granulocyte-macrophage colony stimulating factor. *J. Clin. Invest.* 79:48–51.

Tushinski, R. J., I. T. Oliver, L. J. Guilbert, P. W. Tynan, J. R. Warner, and E. R. Stanley. 1982. Survival of mononuclear phagocytes depends on a lineage-specific growth factor that the differentiated cells selectively destroy. *Cell* 28:71–81.

6. Modulators of CSF Action

Broxmeyer, H. E., L. Juliano, A. Waheed, and R. K. Shadduck. 1985. Release from mouse macrophages of acidic isoferritins that suppress hematopoietic progenitor cells is induced by purified L cell colony stimulating factor and suppressed by human lactoferrin. *J. Cell. Physiol.* 135:3224–3231.

Broxmeyer, H. E., A. Smithyman, R. R. Eger, P. A. Myers, and M. De Sousa. 1978. Identification of lactoferrin as the granulocyte-derived inhibitor of colony-stimulating activity production. *J. Exp. Med.* 148:1052–1067.

Jubinsky, P. T., and E. R. Stanley. 1985. Purification of hemopoietin I: A multilineage hemopoietic growth factor. *Proc. Natl. Acad. Sci. (USA)* 82:2764–2768.

Lord, B. I. 1986. Interactions of regulatory factors in the control of haemopoietic stem cell proliferation. In *Biological Regulation of Cell Proliferation*, ed. R. Baserga, P. Foa, D. Metcalf, and E. E. Polli. New York: Raven Press, pp. 167–177.

Metcalf, D., and S. Russell. 1976. Inhibition by mouse serum of hemopoietic colony formation in vitro. *Exp. Hematol.* 4:339–353.

Paukovits, W. R., O. D. Laerum, and M. Guigon. 1986. Isolation, characterization and synthesis of a chalone-like hemoregulatory peptide. In *Biological Regulation of Cell Proliferation*, ed. R. Baserga, P. Foa, D. Metcalf, and E. E. Polli. New York: Raven Press, pp. 111–119.

Pelus, L. M., H. E. Broxmeyer, J. I. Kurland, and M. A. S. Moore. 1979. Regulation of macrophage and granulocyte proliferation: Specificities of prostaglandin E and lactoferrin. *J. Exp. Med.* 150:277–292.

Stanley, E. R., A. Bartocci, D. Patinkin, M. Rosendaal, and T. R. Bradley.

1986. Regulation of very primitive, multipotent hemopoietic cells by hemopoietin-1. *Cell* 45:667–674.

7. *Actions of the CSFs In Vivo*

Donahue, R. E., E. A. Wang, D. Stone, R. Kamen, G. G. Wong, P. K. Sehgal, D. G. Nathan, and S. C. Clark. 1986. Stimulation of haematopoiesis in primates by continuous infusion of recombinant human GM-CSF. *Nature* 321:872–875.

Kindler, V., B. Thorens, S. De Kossodo, B. Allet, J. F. Eliason, D. Thatcher, N. Farber, and P. Vassalli. 1986. Stimulation of hematopoiesis in vivo by recombinant bacterial murine interleukin 3. *Proc. Natl. Acad. Sci. (USA)* 83:1001–1005.

Metcalf, D., C. G. Begley, G. R. Johnson, N. A. Nicola, A. F. Lopez, and D. J. Williamson. 1986. Effects of purified bacterially-synthesized murine Multi-CSF (IL-3) on hemopoiesis in normal adult mice. *Blood* 68:46–57.

Metcalf, D., C. G. Begley, D. J. Williamson, E. C. Nice, J. DeLamarter, J.-J. Mermod, D. Thatcher, and A. Schmidt. 1987. Hemopoietic responses in mice injected with purified recombinant murine GM-CSF. *Exp. Hematol.* 15:1–9.

Welte, K., M. A. Bonilla, A. P. Gillio, T. C. Boone, G. K. Potter, J. L. Gabrilove, M. A. S. Moore, R. J. O'Reilly, and L. M. Souza. 1987. Recombinant human granulocyte-colony-stimulating factor: Effects on hematopoiesis in normal and cyclophosphamide-treated primates. *J. Exp. Med.* 165:941–948.

8. *Role of the CSFs in Resistance to Infections*

See the suggested readings for Chapters 4 and 7. No publications are in print yet on the effects of CSFs in experimental infections.

9. *Toxic Effects of the CSFs*

Lang, R. A., D. Metcalf, R. A. Cuthbertson, I. Lyons, A. Kelso, G. Kannourakis, J. Williamson, G. Klintworth, T. Gonda, and A. R. Dunn. 1987. Transgenic mice expressing a hemopoietic growth factor gene (GM-CSF) develop an accumulation of activated macrophages, blindness and a fatal syndrome of tissue damage. *Cell* 51:675–686.

Ross, R., E. W. Raines, and D. F. Bowen-Pope. 1986. The biology of platelet-derived growth factor. *Cell* 46:155–169.

10. *Role of the CSFs in Myeloid Leukemia*

Begley, C. G., D. Metcalf, and N. A. Nicola. 1987. Primary human myeloid leukemia cells: Comparative responsiveness to proliferative stimulation by GM-CSF or G-CSF and membrane expression of CSF receptors. *Leukemia* 1:1–8.

Cook, W. D., D. Metcalf, N. A. Nicola, A. W. Burgess, and F. Walker. 1985. Malignant transformation of a growth factor-dependent myloid cell line by Abelson virus without evidence of an autocrine mechanism. *Cell* 41:677–683.

Coulombel, L., C. Eaves, D. Kalousek, and A. Eaves. 1985. Long-term marrow culture of cells from patients with acute myelogenous leukemia: Selection in favor of normal phenotypes in some but not all cases. *J. Clin. Invest.* 75:961–969.

Hozumi, M. 1983. Fundamentals of chemotherapy of myeloid leukemia by induction of leukemia cell differentiation. *Ad. Cancer Res.* 38:121–169.

Lang, R. A., D. Metcalf, N. M. Gough, A. R. Dunn, and T. J. Gonda. 1985. Expression of a hematopoietic growth factor cDNA in a factor-dependent cell line results in autonomous growth and tumorigenicity. *Cell* 43:531–542.

Le Beau, M. M., C. A. Westbrook, M. O. Diaz, R. A. Larson, D. J. Rowley, J. C. Gasson, D. W. Golde, and C. J. Sherr. 1986. Evidence for the involvement of GM-CSF and FMS in the deletion (5q) in myeloid disorders. *Science* 231:984–987.

Metcalf, D. 1980. Clonal extinction of myelomonocytic leukemic cells by serum from mice injected with endotoxin. *Int. J. Cancer* 25:225–233.

———. 1982. Regulator-induced suppression of myelomonocytic leukemic cells: Clonal analysis of early cellular events. *Int. J. Cancer* 30:203–210.

Moore, M. A. S. 1975. In vitro studies in the myeloid leukemias. In *Advances in Acute Leukemia*, ed. F. J. Cleton, D. Crowther, and J. B. Malpas. Amsterdam: North-Holland, pp. 161–227.

Moore, M. A. S., N. Williams, and D. Metcalf. 1973. In vitro colony formation by normal and leukemic human hematopoietic cells: Characterization of colony forming cells. *J. Natl. Cancer Instit.* 50:603–623.

Nicola, N. A., C. G. Begley, and D. Metcalf. 1985. Identification of the human analogue of a regulator that induces differentiation in murine leukaemic cells. *Nature* 314:625–628.

Nicola, N. A., and D. Metcalf. 1986. The colony-stimulating factors and myeloid leukaemia. *Cancer Surveys* 4:789–815.

Pierce, J. H., P. P. De Fiore, S. A. Aaronson, M. Potter, J. Pumphrey, A. Scott, and J. N. Ihle. 1985. Neoplastic transformation of mast cells by Abelson MuLV: Abrogation of IL-3 dependence by a nonautocrine mechanism. *Cell* 41:685–693.

Sachs, L. 1987. Cell differentiation and bypassing of genetic defects in the suppression of malignancy. *Cancer Research* 47:1981–1986.

Upton, A. C., V. K. Jenkins, H. E. Walburg, R. L. Tyndall, J. W. Conklin, and N. Wald. 1966. Observations on viral-, chemical- and radiation-induced myeloid leukemia and lymphoid leukemias of Rf mice. *Natl. Cancer Instit. Monograph* 22:329–347.

Young, D. C., and J. D. Griffin. 1986. Autocrine secretion of GM-CSF in acute myeloblastic leukemia. *Blood* 68:1178–1181.

Credits

The author is indebted to the publishers of the following publications for permission to reproduce the figures and tables listed below.

Figure 10. Reproduced from D. Metcalf, *The Hemopoietic Colony Stimulating Factors* (Amsterdam: Elsevier, 1984).

Figure 13. Reproduced from D. Metcalf, "The granulocyte-macrophage colony stimulating factors," *Science* 229:16–22, 1985. Copyright © American Association for the Advancement of Science.

Figure 14. Reproduced from N. A. Nicola and D. Metcalf, "Binding of ^{125}I-labeled granulocyte colony-stimulating factor to normal murine hemopoietic cells," *J. Cell. Physiol.* 124:313–321, 1985.

Figure 17. Reproduced from D. Metcalf, *The Hemopoietic Colony Stimulating Factors* (Amsterdam: Elsevier, 1984).

Figure 18. Reproduced from D. Metcalf, "The molecular control of normal and leukaemic granulocytes and macrophages," *Proc. R. Soc. Lond. (B)* 230:389–423, 1987.

Figure 19. Reproduced from D. Metcalf, "Clonal analysis of proliferation and differentiation of paired daughter cells: Action of granulocyte-macrophage colony-stimulating factor on granulocyte-macrophage precursors," *Proc. Natl. Acad. Sci. (U.S.A.)* 77:5327–5330, 1980.

Figure 20. Reproduced from D. Metcalf, "The molecular control of normal and leukaemic granulocytes and macrophages," *Proc. R. Soc. Lond. (B)* 230:389–423, 1987.

Figure 31. Reproduced from D. Metcalf, "The molecular control of normal and leukaemic granulocytes and macrophages," *Proc. R. Soc. Lond. (B)* 230:389–423, 1987.

Figure 32. Reproduced from D. Metcalf, C. G. Begley, D. J. Williamson, E. C. Nice, J. DeLamarter, J. J. Mermod, D. Thatcher, and A. Schmidt, "Hemopoietic responses in mice injected with purified recombinant murine GM-CSF," *Exp. Hematol.* 15:1–9, 1987.

Figure 34. Reproduced from D. Metcalf, "The molecular control of normal and leukaemic granulocytes and macrophages," *Proc. R. Soc. Lond. (B)* 230:389–423, 1987.

Figure 35. Reproduced from D. Metcalf, "The molecular control of normal and leukaemic granulocytes and macrophages," *Proc. R. Soc. Lond. (B)* 230:389–423, 1987.

Figure 40. Reproduced from D. Metcalf, "The granulocyte-macrophage colony stimulating factors," *Science* 229:16–22, 1985. Copyright © American Association for the Advancement of Science.

Figure 43. Reproduced from C. G. Begley, D. Metcalf, and N. A. Nicola, "Primary human myeloid leukemic cells: Comparative responsiveness to proliferative stimulation by GM-CSF or G-CSF and membrane expression of CSF receptors," *Leukemia* 1:1–8, 1987. Copyright © Williams & Wilkins.

Tables 3 and 4. Adapted from N. A. Nicola, "Why do hemopoietic growth factor receptors interact with each other?" *Immunology Today* 8:134–140, 1987.

Index